FIRST AID FOR THE®

Obstetrics & Gynecology Clerkship

Second Edition

LATHA G. STEAD, MD
Associate Professor of Emergency Medicine
Mayo Clinic College of Medicine
Rochester, Minnesota

S. MATTHEW STEAD, MD, PhD
Assistant Professor of Neurology
Mayo Clinic College of Medicine
Rochester, Minnesota

MATTHEW S. KAUFMAN, MD
Fellow in Hematology
Long Island Jewish Medical Center
Albert Einstein College of Medicine
New Hyde Park, New York

LUIS F. SUAREZ, MD
Chief Resident in Obstetrics and Gynecology
Mayo Graduate School of Medicine
Rochester, Minnesota

D0206454

McGraw-Hill
MEDICAL PUBLISHING DIVISION

New York / Chicago / San Francisco / Lisbon / London / Madrid / Mexico City
Milan / New Delhi / San Juan / Seoul / Singapore / Sydney / Toronto

First Aid for the® Obstetrics & Gynecology Clerkship, Second Edition

1 2 3 4 5 6 7 8 9 0 QPD/QPD 0 9 8 7 6

ISBN-13: 978-0-07-144874-1
ISBN-10: 0-07-144874-8

Notice

Medicine is an ever-changing science. As new research and clinical experience broaden our knowledge, changes in treatment and drug therapy are required. The authors and the publisher of this work have checked with sources believed to be reliable in their efforts to provide information that is complete and generally in accord with the standards accepted at the time of publication. However, in view of the possibility of human error or changes in medical sciences, neither the authors nor the publisher nor any other party who has been involved in the preparation or publication of this work warrants that the information contained herein is in every respect accurate or complete, and they disclaim all responsibility for any errors or omissions or for the results obtained from use of the information contained in this work. Readers are encouraged to confirm the information contained herein with other sources. For example and in particular, readers are advised to check the product information sheet included in the package of each drug they plan to administer to be certain that the information contained in this work is accurate and that changes have not been made in the recommended dose or in the contraindications for administration. This recommendation is of particular importance in connection with new or infrequently used drugs.

This book was set in Electra LH by Rainbow Graphics.
The editor was Catherine A. Johnson.
The production supervisor was Catherine Saggese.
Project management was provided by Rainbow Graphics.
Quebecor World Dubuque was the printer and binder.

This book is printed on acid-free paper.

Library of Congress Cataloging-in-Publication Data

Stead, Latha G.
    First aid for the obstetrics & gynecology clerkship : the student to student guide / Latha G.
Stead, S. Matthew Stead, Matthew S. Kaufman. – 2nd ed.
      p. ; cm.
    Rev. ed. of: First aid for the obstetrics and gynecology clerkship / authors, Robert Feig,
Nicole Collette Johnson. 2001
    Includes index.
    ISBN 0-07-144874-8
      1. Obstetrics–Study and teaching (Graduate) 2. Gynecology–Study and teaching (Graduate)
    3. Clinical medicine–Study and teaching (Graduate) I. Stead, S. Matthew. II. Kaufman, Matthew S.
    III. Feig, Robert. First aid for the obstetrics and gynecology clerkship.
      [DNLM: 1. Clinical Clerkship. 2. Obstetrics. 3. Gynecology. WQ 18 S799f2006]
    RG141.F45 2006
    618.0076–dc22

                                                                                2006046596

International Edition ISBN-13: 978-0-07-110092-2; ISBN-10: 0-07-110092-X
Copyright © 2007. Exclusive rights by The McGraw-Hill Companies, Inc. for manufacture and export. This book cannot be re-exported from the country to which it is consigned by McGraw-Hill. The International Edition is not available in North America.

STUDENT AND RESIDENT REVIEWERS

NICHOLAS KONGOASA, MBBS
Class of 2005
Manchester University School of Medicine
Manchester, United Kingdom

ANJULIE GANTI, MSW
MPH Candidate
Columbia University
New York, New York

SARAH HARPER, MD
Resident in Internal Medicine
The George Washington University School
    of Medicine
Washington, District of Columbia
Class of 2005
University of Pittsburgh School of Medicine

HOWARD K. MELL, MD, MPH
Resident in Emergency Medicine
Mayo Graduate School of Medicine
Rochester, Minnesota

SAILAJA ENDURI, MBBS
Research Trainee
Department of Emergency Medicine
Mayo Clinic
Rochester, Minnesota

SEAN SMITH
Class of 2007
Mayo Clinic College of Medicine
Rochester, Minnesota

VIPUL PATEL, MD
Resident in Orthopedics
New York University
New York, New York

LEKSHMI VAIDYANATHAN, MBBS
Research Trainee
Department of Emergency Medicine
Mayo Clinic
Rochester, Minnesota

ASHWINI SAGAR
Class of 2007
UCLA School of Medicine
Los Angeles, California

BENJAMIN J. SANDEFUR
Class of 2008
Mayo Clinic College of Medicine
Rochester, Minnesota

GITA THANARAJASINGHAM
Class of 2008
Mayo Clinic College of Medicine
Rochester, Minnesota

CONTENTS

Introduction   vii

Acknowledgments   ix

How to Contribute   xi

SECTION I: HOW TO SUCCEED IN THE OBSTETRICS & GYNECOLOGY CLERKSHIP   **1**

SECTION II: HIGH-YIELD FACTS IN OBSTETRICS   **11**

Normal Anatomy   13

Diagnosis of Pregnancy   19

Physiology of Pregnancy   23

Antepartum   43

Intrapartum   57

Postpartum   87

Medical Conditions and Infections in Pregnancy   97

Complications of Pregnancy   115

Spontaneous Abortion, Ectopic Pregnancy, and Fetal Death   135

Induced Abortion   147

SECTION III: HIGH-YIELD FACTS IN GYNECOLOGY   **151**

Contraception and Sterilization   153

Infertility   163

Menstruation   169

Abnormal Uterine Bleeding   179

Pelvic Pain   183

Endometriosis and Adenomyosis   187

Pelvic Masses   191

Cervical Dysplasia   197

Cervical Cancer   203

Endometrial Cancer   211

Ovarian Cancer   217

Vulvar Dysplasia and Cancer   225

Gestational Trophoblastic Neoplasia   229

Sexually Transmitted Diseases and Vaginitis   235

Vulvar Disorders   245

Menopause   249

Pelvic Relaxation   255

Women's Health   261

SECTION IV: **CLASSIFIED**   **275**

Awards and Opportunities   276

Web Sites of Interest   278

Index   281

INTRODUCTION

This clinical study aid was designed in the tradition of the *First Aid* series of books, formatted in the same way as the other titles in this series. Topics are listed by bold headings to the left, while the "meat" of the topic comprises the middle column. The outside margins contain mnemonics, diagrams, summary or warning statements, "pearls," and other memory aids. These are further classified as "exam tip" noted by the ⬛ symbol, "ward tip" noted by the ⬛ symbol, and "typical scenario" noted by the ⬛ symbol.

The content of this book is based on the American Professors of Gynecology and Obstetrics (APGO) and the American College of Obstetricians and Gynecologists (ACOG) recommendations for the OB/GYN curriculum for third-year medical students. Each of the chapters contain the major topics central to the practice of obstetrics and gynecology and closely parallel APGO's medical student learning objectives. This book also targets the obstetrics and gynecology content on the USMLE Step 2 examination.

The OB/GYN clerkship can be an exciting hands-on experience. You will get to deliver babies, assist in surgeries, and see patients in the clinic setting. You will find that rather than simply preparing you for the success on the clerkship exam, this book will also help guide you in the clinical diagnosis and treatment of the many interesting problems you will see during your obstetrics and gynecology rotation.

ACKNOWLEDGMENTS

We would like to thank the following faculty for their help in reviewing the manuscript for the first edition of this book:

Eugene C. Toy, MD
Academic Chief and Program Director
Obstetrics-Gynecology Residency
The Methodist Hospital
Houston, Texas

Patti Jayne Ross, MD
Clerkship Director
Department of Obstetrics and Gynecology
The University of Texas–Houston Medical School
Houston, Texas

HOW TO CONTRIBUTE

To continue to produce a high-yield review source for the obstetrics and gynecology clerkship, you are invited to submit any suggestions or correction. Please send us your suggestions for:

- New facts, mnemonics, diagrams, and illustrations
- Low-yield facts to remove

For each entry incorporated into the next edition, you will receive personal acknowledgment. Diagrams, tables, partial entries, updates, corrections, and study hints are also appreciated, and significant contributions will be compensated at the discretion of the authors. Also let us know about material in this edition that you feel is low yield and should be deleted. You are also welcome to send general comments and feedback, although due to the volume of e-mails, we may not be able to respond to each of these.

The **preferred way** to submit entries, suggestions, or corrections is via **electronic mail**. Please include name, address, school affiliation, phone number, and e-mail address (if different from the address of origin). If there are multiple entries, please consolidate into a single e-mail or file attachment. Please send submissions to:

firstaidclerkships@gmail.com

Otherwise, please send entries, neatly written or typed or on disk (Microsoft Word) to:

Latha G. Stead, MD
C/o Catherine A. Johnson
Senior Editor
McGraw-Hill Medical
Two Penn Plaza, 11th Floor
New York, NY 10121

All entries become property of the authors and are subject to editing and reviewing. Please verify all data and spellings carefully. In the event that similar or duplicate entries are received, only the first entry received will be used. Include a reference to a standard textbook to facilitate verification of the fact. Please follow the style, punctuation, and format of this edition if possible.

How to Succeed in the Obstetrics & Gynecology Clerkship

How to Behave on the Wards	2
How to Organize Your Learning	5
How to Prepare for the Clinical Clerkship and USMLE Step 2 Exam	5
Terminology	7
Sample Obstetric Admission History and Physical	7
Sample Delivery Note	9
Sample Postpartum Note	9
Sample Post-NSVD Discharge Orders	10
Sample Post–Cesarean Section Note	10
Sample Discharge Orders Post–Cesarean Section	10

Be on Time

Most OB/GYN teams begin rounding between 6 and 7 A.M. If you are expected to "pre-round," you should give yourself at least 10 minutes per patient that you are following to see the patient and learn about the events that occurred overnight. Like all working professionals, you will face occasional obstacles to punctuality, but make sure this is occasional. When you first start a rotation, try to show up at least 15 minutes early until you get the routine figured out.

Dress in a Professional Manner

Even if the resident wears scrubs and the attending wears stiletto heels, you must dress in a professional, conservative manner. Wear a *short* white coat over your clothes unless discouraged (as in pediatrics).

> **Men** should wear long pants, with cuffs covering the ankle, a long collared shirt, and a tie. No jeans, no sneakers, no short-sleeved shirts.
> **Women** should wear long pants or knee-length skirt, blouse or dressy sweater. No jeans, no sneakers, no heels greater than 1½ inches, no open-toed shoes.
> **Both men and women** may wear scrubs occasionally, during overnight call or in the operating room or birthing ward. Do not make this your uniform.

Act in a Pleasant Manner

The rotation is often difficult, stressful, and tiring. You will have a smoother experience if you are nice to be around. Smile a lot and learn everyone's name. If you do not understand or disagree with a treatment plan or diagnosis, do not "challenge." Instead, say "I'm sorry, I don't quite understand, could you please explain . . ."

Try to look interested to attendings and residents. Sometimes this stuff is boring, or sometimes you're not in the mood. However, when someone is trying to teach you something, look grateful and not tortured.

Always treat patients professionally and with respect. This is crucial to practicing good medicine, but on a less important level if a resident or attending spots you being impolite or unprofessional, it will damage your grade and evaluation quicker than any dumb answer on rounds ever could. And be nice to the nurses. Really nice. Learn names; bring back pens and food from pharmaceutical lunches and give them out. If they like you, they can make your life a lot easier and make you look good in front of the residents and attendings.

Be Aware of the Hierarchy

The way in which this will affect you will vary from hospital to hospital and team to team, but it is always present to some degree. In general, address your questions regarding ward functioning to interns or residents. Address your medical questions to attendings; make an effort to be somewhat informed on your subject prior to asking attendings medical questions. But please don't ask a question just to transparently show off what you know. It's annoying to everyone. Show off by seeming interested and asking real questions that you have when they come up.

Address Patients and Staff in a Respectful Way

Address patients as Sir or Ma'am, or Mr., Mrs., or Miss. Try not to address patients as "honey," "sweetie," and the like. Although you may feel these names are friendly, patients will think you have forgotten their name, that you are being inappropriately familiar, or both. Address all physicians as "doctor," unless told otherwise.

Be Helpful to Your Residents

Being helpful involves taking responsibility for patients that you've been assigned to, and even for some that you haven't. If you've been assigned to a patient, know everything there is to know about her, her history, test results, details about her medical problems, and prognosis. Keep your interns or residents informed of new developments that they might not be aware of, and ask them for any updates as well.

If you have the opportunity to make a resident look good, take it. If some new complication comes up with a patient, tell the resident about it before the attending gets a chance to grill the resident on it. And don't hesitate to give credit to a resident for some great teaching in front of an attending. These things make the resident's life easier, and he or she will be grateful and the rewards will come your way.

Volunteer to do things that will help out. So what if you have to run to the lab to follow up on a stat H&H? It helps everybody out, and it is appreciated. Observe and anticipate. If a resident is always hunting around for some tape to do a dressing change every time you round on a particular patient, get some tape ahead of time.

Respect Patients' Rights

1. All patients have the right to have their personal medical information kept private. This means do not discuss the patient's information with family members without that patient's consent and do not discuss any patient in hallways, elevators, or cafeterias.
2. All patients have the right to refuse treatment. This means they can refuse treatment by a specific individual (you, the medical student) or of a specific type (Pap smear). Patients can even refuse lifesaving treatment. The only exceptions to this rule are a patient who is deemed to not have the capacity to make decisions or understand situations—in which case a health care proxy should be sought—or a patient who is suicidal or homicidal.
3. All patients should be informed of the right to seek advanced directives on admission. This is often done by the admissions staff, in a booklet. If your patient is chronically ill or has a life-threatening illness, address the subject of advance directives with the assistance of your attending.

Volunteer More

Be self-propelled. Volunteer to help with a procedure or a difficult task. Volunteer to give a talk on a topic of your choice. Ask your resident about the length and timing of the talk. Volunteer to take additional patients. Volunteer to stay late. The more unpleasant the task, the better.

Be a Team Player

Help other medical students with their tasks; teach them information you have learned. Support your supervising intern or resident whenever possible. Never steal the spotlight, steal a procedure, or make a fellow medical student look bad.

Be Honest

If you don't understand, don't know, or didn't do it, make sure you always say that. Never say or document information that is false (for example, don't say "bowel sounds normal" when you did not listen).

Keep Patient Information Handy

Use a clipboard, notebook, or index cards to keep patient information, including a miniature history and physical, lab, and test results at hand.

Present Patient Information in an Organized Manner

Here is a template for the "bullet" presentation:

> "This is a **[age]**-year-old **[gender]** with a history of **[major history such as abdominal surgery, pertinent OB/GYN history]** who presented on **[date]** with **[major symptoms, such as pelvic pain, fever]**, and was found to have **[working diagnosis]**. **[Tests done]** showed **[results]**. Yesterday the patient **[state important changes, new plan, new tests, new medications]**. This morning the patient feels **[state the patient's words]**, and the physical exam is significant for **[state major findings]**. Plan is **[state plan]**.

The newly admitted patient generally deserves a longer presentation following the complete history and physical format (see below).

Some patients have extensive histories. The whole history can and probably should be present in the admission note, but in ward presentation it is often too much to absorb. In these cases, it will be very much appreciated by your team if you can generate a good summary that maintains an accurate picture of the patient. This usually takes some thought, but it's worth it.

Document Information in an Organized Manner

A complete medical student initial history and physical is neat, legible, organized, and usually two to three pages long (see page 7).

The main advantage to doing the OB/GYN clerkship is that you get to see patients. The patient is the key to learning and the source of most satisfaction and frustration on the wards. One enormously helpful tip is to try to skim this book before starting your rotation. Starting OB/GYN can make you feel like you're in a foreign land, and all that studying the first two years doesn't help much. You have to start from scratch in some ways, and it will help enormously if you can skim through this book before you start. Get some of the terminology straight, get some of the major points down, and it won't seem so strange.

Select Your Study Material

We recommend:
- This review book, *First Aid for the® Obstetrics & Gynecology Clerkship*, 2nd edition
- A full-text online journal database, such as *www.mdconsult.com* (subscription is $99/year for students)
- A small pocket reference book to look up lab values, clinical pathways, and the like, such as *Maxwell Quick Medical Reference* (ISBN 0964519119, $7)
- A small book to look up drugs, such as *Pocket Pharmacopoeia* (Tarascon Publishers, $8)

As You See Patients, Note Their Major Symptoms and Diagnosis for Review

Your reading on the symptom-based topics above should be done with a specific patient in mind. For example, if a postmenopausal patient comes to the office with increasing abdominal girth and is thought to have ovarian cancer, read about ovarian cancer in the review book that night.

Prepare a Talk on a Topic

You may be asked to give a small talk once or twice during your rotation. If not, you should volunteer! Feel free to choose a topic that is on your list; however, realize that this may be considered dull by the people who hear the lecture. The ideal topic is slightly uncommon but not rare. To prepare a talk on a topic, read about it in a major textbook and a review article not more than two years old, and then search online or in the library for recent developments or changes in treatment.

HOW TO PREPARE FOR THE CLINICAL CLERKSHIP AND USMLE STEP 2 EXAM

If you have read about your core illnesses and core symptoms, you will know a great deal about medicine. To study for the clerkship exam, we recommend:

2–3 weeks before exam: Read this entire review book, taking notes.
10 days before exam: Read the notes you took during the rotation on your core content list and the corresponding review book sections.

5 days before exam: Read this entire review book, concentrating on lists and mnemonics.

2 days before exam: Exercise, eat well, skim the book, and go to bed early.

1 day before exam: Exercise, eat well, review your notes and the mnemonics, and go to bed on time. Do not have any caffeine after 2 P.M.

Other helpful studying strategies include:

Study with Friends

Group studying can be very helpful. Other people may point out areas that you have not studied enough and may help you focus on the goal. If you tend to get distracted by other people in the room, limit this to less than half of your study time.

Study in a Bright Room

Find the room in your house or in your library that has the best, brightest light. This will help prevent you from falling asleep. If you don't have a bright light, get a halogen desk lamp or a light that simulates sunlight (not a tanning lamp).

Eat Light, Balanced Meals

Make sure your meals are balanced, with lean protein, fruits and vegetables, and fiber. A high-sugar, high-carbohydrate meal will give you an initial burst of energy for 1–2 hours, but then you'll drop.

Take Practice Exams

The point of practice exams is not so much the content that is contained in the questions but the training of sitting still for 3 hours and trying to pick the best answer for each and every question.

Tips for Answering Questions

All questions are intended to have one best answer. When answering questions, follow these guidelines:

Read the answers first. For all questions longer than two sentences, reading the answers first can help you sift through the question for the key information.

Look for the words "EXCEPT," "MOST," "LEAST," "NOT," "BEST," "WORST," "TRUE," "FALSE," "CORRECT," "INCORRECT," "ALWAYS," and "NEVER." If you find one of these words, circle or underline it for later comparison with the answer.

Evaluate each answer as being either true or false. Example:
Which of the following is *least* likely to be associated with pelvic pain?
A. endometriosis **T**
B. ectopic pregnancy **T**

C. ovarian cancer **F**
D. ovarian torsion **T**

By comparing the question, noting LEAST, to the answers, "C" is the best answer.

TERMINOLOGY

G (gravidity) 3 = total number of pregnancies, including normal and abnormal intrauterine pregnancies, abortions, ectopic pregnancies, and hydatidiform moles (*Remember, if patient was pregnant with twins, G = 1.*)
P (parity) 3 = number of deliveries > 500 grams or ≥ 20 weeks' gestation, stillborn (dead) or alive (*Remember, if patient was pregnant with twins, P = 1.*)
Ab (abortus) 0 = number of pregnancies that were lost before the 20th gestational week or in which the fetus weighs < 500 grams
LC (living children) 3 = number of successful pregnancy outcomes (*Remember, if patient was pregnant with twins, LC = 2.*)

Or use the "TPAL" system if it is used at your medical school:

T = number of term deliveries (3)
P = number of preterm deliveries (0)
A = number of abortions (0)
L = number of living children (3)

SAMPLE OBSTETRIC ADMISSION HISTORY AND PHYSICAL

Date
Time
Identification: 25 yo G3P2
Estimated gestational age (EGA): $38^{5}/_{7}$ weeks
Last menstrual period (LMP): First day of LMP
Estimated date of confinement: Due date (*specify how it was determined*) by LMP or by _____ wk US (*Sonograms are most accurate for dating EGA when done at < 20 weeks.*)
Chief complaint (CC): Uterine contractions (UCs) q 7 min since 0100
History of present illness (HPI): 25 yo G3P2 with an intrauterine pregnancy (IUP) at $38^{5}/_{7}$ wks GA, well dated by LMP (10/13/05) and US at 10 weeks GA, who presented to L&D with CC of uterine contractions q 7 min. Prenatal care (PNC) at Montefiore Hospital (12 visits, first visit at 7 wks GA), uterine size = to dates, prenatal BP range 100–126/64–83. Problem list includes H/o + group B *Streptococcus* (GBS) and a +PPD with subsequent negative chest x-ray in 5/06. Pt admitted in early active labor with a vaginal exam (VE) 4/90/–2.

Past Obstetric History
'02 NSVD @ term, girl, wt 3,700 g
No complications during pregnancy, delivery, and puerperium
No developmental problem in child

'04 NSVD @ term, boy, wt 3,900 g

Postpartum hemorrhage, atonic uterus, syntometrine given and hemorrhage resolved

No developmental problem in child

Past Gynecological History

No significant history of PID, IMB, dyspareunia, postcoital bleed

Last smear: 3/4/05—normal

Contraception: Nil

Blood group: O–, anti D prophylaxis given at 30 weeks GA

Allergies: NKDA

Medications: PNV, Fe

Medical Hx: H/o asthma (asymptomatic × 7 yrs), UTI × 1 @ 30 wks s/p Macrobid 100 mg × 7 d, neg PPD with subsequent neg CXR (5/06)

Surgical Hx: Negative

Social Hx: Negative

Family Hx: Mother—DM II, father—HTN

ROS: Bilateral low back pain

PE

General appearance: Alert and oriented (A&O), no acute distress (NAD)

Vital signs: T, BP, P, R

HEENT: No scleral icterus, pale conjunctiva

Neck: Thyroid midline, no masses, no lymphadenopathy (LAD)

Lungs: CTA bilaterally

Back: No CVA tenderness

Heart: II/VI SEM

Breasts: No masses, symmetric

Abdomen: Gravid, nontender

Fundal height: 36 cm

Estimated fetal weight (EFW): 3,500 g by Leopold's

Presentation: Vertex

Extremities: Mild lower extremity edema, nonpitting

Pelvis: Adequate

VE: Dilatation (4 cm)/effacement (90%)/station (−2); sterile speculum exam (SSE)? (Nitrazine?, Ferning?, Pooling?); membranes intact

US (L&D): Vertex presentation confirmed, anterior placenta, AFI = 13.2

Fetal monitor: Baseline FHR = 150, reactive. Toco = UCs q 5 min

Labs

Blood type: A+

Antibody screen: Neg

Rubella: Immune

HbsAg

VDRL: Nonreactive

FTA

GC

Chlamydia

HIV: See prenatal records

1 hr GTT: 105

3 hr GTT

PPD: + s/p neg CXR

CXR: Neg 5/06

AFP: Neg × 3

Amnio
PAP: NL
Hgb/Hct
Urine: + blood, − protein, − glucose, − nitrite, 2 WBCs
GBS: +

Assessment
1. Intrauterine pregancy @ $38^{5}/_{7}$ wks GA in early active labor
2. Group B strep +
3. H/o + PPD with subsequent − CXR 5/06
4. H/o UTI @ 30 wks GA, s/p Rx—resolved
5. H/o asthma—stable × 7 yrs, no meds

Plan
1. Admit to L&D
2. NPO except ice chips
3. H&H, VDRL, and hold tube
4. D5 LR TRA 125 cc/hr
5. Ampicillin 2 g IV load, then 1 g IV q 4 hrs (for GBS)
6. External fetal monitors (EFMs)
7. Prep and enema

SAMPLE DELIVERY NOTE

Always sign and date your notes.

Normal spontaneous vaginal delivery (NSVD) of viable male infant over an intact perineum @ 12:35 P.M., Apgars 8&9, wt 3,654 g without difficulty. Position LOA, bulb suction, nuchal cord × 1 reducible. Spontaneous delivery of intact 3-vessel cord placenta @ 12:47 P.M., fundal massage and pitocin initiated, fundus firm. 2nd-degree perineal laceration repaired under local anesthesia with 3-0 vicryl. Estimated blood loss (EBL) = 450 cc. Mom and baby stable. Doctors: Mell & Thanarajasingham.

SAMPLE POSTPARTUM NOTE

S: Pt ambulating, voiding, tolerating a regular diet
O: *Vitals*
Heart: RRR without murmurs
Lungs: CTA bilaterally
Breasts: Nonengorged, colostrum expressed bilaterally
Fundus: Firm, mildly tender to palpation, 1 fingerbreadth below umbilicus
Lochia: Moderate amount, rubra
Perineum: Intact, no edema
Extremities: No edema, nontender
Postpartum Hgb: 9.7
VDRL: NR
A: S/p NSVD, PP day # 1—progressing well, afebrile, stable
P: Continue postpartum care

SAMPLE POST-NSVD DISCHARGE ORDERS

1. D/c pt home
2. Pelvic rest × 6 weeks
3. Postpartum check in 4–6 weeks
4. D/c meds: FeSO$_4$ 300 mg 1 tab PO tid, #90 *(For Hgb < 10; opinions vary on when to give FE postpartum)*
   Colace 100 mg 1 tab PO bid PRN no bowel movement, #60

SAMPLE POST–CESAREAN SECTION NOTE

S: Pt c/o abdominal pain, no flatus, minimal ambulation
O: *Vitals*
    I&O (urinary intake and output): Last 8 hrs = 750/695
    Heart: RRR without murmurs
    Lungs: CTA bilaterally
    Breasts: Nonengorged, no colostrum expressed
    Fundus: Firm, tender to palpation, 1 fingerbreadth above umbilicus; incision without erythema/edema; C/D/I (clean/dry/intact); normal abdominal bowel sounds (NABS)
    Lochia: Scant, rubra
    Perineum: Intact, Foley catheter in place
    Extremities: 1+ pitting edema bilateral LEs, nontender
    Postpartum Hgb: 11
    VDRL: NR
A: S/p primary low-transverse c/s secondary to arrest of descent, POD # 1– afebrile, + flatus, stable
P: 1. D/c Foley
    2. Strict I&O—Call HO if UO < 120 cc/4 hrs
    3. Clear liquid diet
    4. Heplock IV once patient tolerates clears
    5. Ambulate qid
    6. Incentive spirometry 10×/hr
    7. Tylenol #3 2 tabs PO q 4 hrs PRN pain

Reporting about flatus and bowel movements is important after a C-section. These are less relevant after an NSVD.

SAMPLE DISCHARGE ORDERS POST–CESAREAN SECTION

1. D/c patient home
2. Pelvic rest × 4 weeks
3. Incision check in 1 week
4. Discharge meds:
   Tylenol #3 1–2 tabs PO q 4 hrs PRN pain, #30
   Colace 100 mg 1 tab PO bid, #60

SECTION II

High-Yield Facts in Obstetrics

▶ Normal Anatomy

▶ Diagnosis of Pregnancy

▶ Physiology of Pregnancy

▶ Antepartum

▶ Intrapartum

▶ Postpartum

▶ Medical Conditions and Infections in Pregnancy

▶ Complications of Pregnancy

▶ Spontaneous Abortion, Ectopic Pregnancy, and Fetal Death

▶ Induced Abortion

HIGH-YIELD FACTS IN

Normal Anatomy

Vulva   14

Vagina   15

Cervix   15

Uterus   15

Ligaments of the Pelvic Viscera   16

Fallopian (Uterine) Tubes   17

Ovaries   17

The vulva consists of the labia majora, labia minora, mons pubis, clitoris, vestibule of the vagina, vestibular bulb, and the greater vestibular glands. Basically, it is the external female genitalia (see Figure 2-1).

Blood Supply

From branches of the external and internal pudendal arteries, which are subdivisions of the hypogastric artery (internal iliac).

Lymph

Medial group of superficial inguinal nodes.

Nerve Supply

- **Pudendal branches:**
  - **Anterior parts of vulva:** Ilioinguinal nerves and the genital branch of the genitofemoral nerves.
  - **Posterior parts:** Perineal nerves and posterior cutaneous nerves of the thigh.

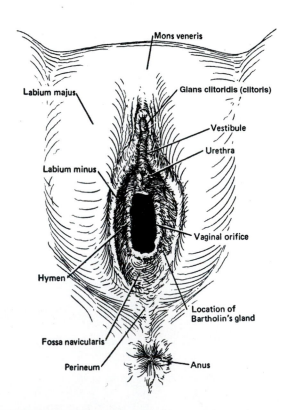

FIGURE 2-1. External female genitalia.

(Reproduced, with permission, from Pernoll ML. *Handbook of Obstetrics and Gynecology*, 10th ed. New York: McGraw-Hill, 2001: 22.)

Blood Supply

- **Hypogastric artery (anastomotic network):**
  - **Vaginal branch of the uterine artery** is the primary supply of the vagina.
  - **Middle rectal and inferior vaginal branches of the hypogastric artery** (internal iliac artery) are secondary blood supplies.
- Anastomoses with cervical arteries.

Nerve Supply

- **Hypogastric plexus:** Sympathetic innervation
- **Pelvic nerve:** Parasympathetic innervation

Components

- **Portio vaginalis:** Portion of the cervix projecting into the vagina
- **External os:** Lowermost opening of the cervix into the vagina
- **Ectocervix:** Portion of the cervix exterior to the external os
- **Endocervical canal:** Passageway between the external os and the uterus
- **Internal os:** Uppermost opening of the cervix into the uterine cavity

Cervical Epithelium

The cervix is covered by both **columnar** and **stratified nonkeratinizing squamous** epithelia. The **squamocolumnar junction,** where these two meet, is the most important cytologic and colposcopic landmark, as this is where over 90% of lower genital tract neoplasias arise.

Blood Supply

Cervical and vaginal branch of the uterine artery, which arises from the internal iliac artery.

Nerve Supply

Hypogastric plexus.

Components

- **Fundus:** Uppermost region of uterus
- **Corpus:** Body of the uterus
- **Cornu:** Part of uterus that joins the fallopian tubes
- **Cervix:** Inferior part of the uterus that connects to the vagina
  - **Internal os:** Opening of cervix on the uterine side
  - **External os:** Opening of cervix on the vaginal side
  - **Cervical canal:** Connects the vagina and the endometrium

Histology

- **Mesometrium:** The visceral peritoneum reflects against the uterus and forms this outermost layer of the organ (the side that faces the viscera).
- **Myometrium:** The smooth muscle layer of uterus. It has three parts:
  1. Outer longitudinal
  2. Middle oblique
  3. Inner longitudinal
- **Endometrium:** The mucosal layer of the uterus, made up of columnar epithelium, 1–6 mm.

Blood Supply

- **Uterine arteries:** Arise from hypogastric artery (internal iliac artery)
- **Ovarian arteries**

Nerve Supply

- **Superior hypogastric plexus**
- **Inferior hypogastric plexus**
- **Common iliac nerves**

LIGAMENTS OF THE PELVIC VISCERA

- **Broad ligament:** Peritoneal fold extends from the lateral pelvic wall to the uterus and adnexa. Contains the fallopian (uterine) tube, round ligament, uterine and ovarian blood vessels, lymph, ureterovaginal nerves, and ureter (see Figure 2-2).

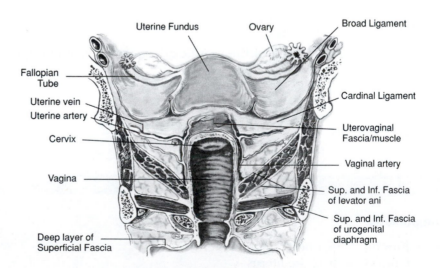

FIGURE 2-2. Supporting structures of the pelvic viscera.

(Reproduced, with permission, from Lindarkis NM, Lott S. *Digging Up the Bones: Obstetrics and Gynecology.* New York: McGraw-Hill, 1998: 2.)

HIGH-YIELD FACTS

Normal Anatomy

- **Round ligament:** The remains of the gubernaculum; extends from the corpus of the uterus down and laterally through the inguinal canal and terminates in the labia majora.
- **Cardinal ligament:** Extends from the cervix and lateral vagina to the pelvic wall; functions to support the uterus.
- **Uterosacral ligaments:** Each ligament extends from an attachment posterolaterally to the supravaginal portion of the cervix and inserts into the fascia over the sacrum.

FALLOPIAN (UTERINE) TUBES

The fallopian tubes extend from the superior lateral aspects of the uterus through the superior fold of the broad ligament laterally to the ovaries.

Parts, from Lateral to Medial

- **Infundibulum:** The lateralmost part the uterine tube. The free edge is connected to the fimbriae.
- **Ampulla:** Widest section.
- **Isthmus:** Narrowest part.
- **Intramural part:** Pierces uterine wall.

Blood Supply

From uterine and ovarian arteries.

Nerve Supply

Pelvic plexus (autonomic) and ovarian plexus.

OVARIES

The ovaries lie on the posterior aspect of the broad ligament, and are attached to the broad ligament by the mesovarium. They are not covered by peritoneum.

Blood Supply

Ovarian artery, which arises from the aorta at the level of L1. Veins drain into the vena cava on the right side and the renal vein on the left.

Nerve Supply

Derived from the aortic plexus.

Histology

Ovaries are covered by tunica albuginea, a fibrous capsule. The tunica albuginea is covered by germinal epithelium.

Diagnosis of Pregnancy

β-hCG   21

Fetal Heart Tones (FHTs)   22

Ultrasonic Scanning (US)   22

Some women experience vaginal bleeding early in pregnancy, and therefore fail to recognize their condition.

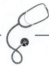

Nausea and/or vomiting occurs in approximately 70–85% of pregnancies, most notably at 2–12 weeks' GA, and typically in the A.M.

Hyperemesis gravidarum is frequent vomiting that typically occurs early in pregnancy. When severe, it can result in weight loss, dehydration, acidosis (from starvation), alkalosis (from loss of HCl in vomitus), and hypokalemia.

History

The majority of women have amenorrhea from the last menstrual period (LMP) until after the birth of their baby.

Symptoms

Although not specific to pregnancy, these symptoms may alert the patient to the fact that she is pregnant:

- Breast enlargement and tenderness from about 6 weeks' gestational age (GA).
- Areolar enlargement and increased pigmentation after 6 weeks' GA.
- Colostrum secretion may begin after 16 weeks' GA.
- Nausea with or without vomiting, from about the date of the missed period.
- Urinary frequency, nocturia, and bladder irritability due to increased bladder circulation and pressure from the enlarging uterus.

Signs

Some clinical signs can be noted, but may be difficult to quantify:

- Breast enlargement, tension, and venous distention—particularly obvious in the primigravida.
- Bimanual examination reveals a soft, cystic, globular uterus with enlargement consistent with the duration of pregnancy (see Table 3-1).
- **Chadwick's sign:** Bluish discoloration of vagina and cervix, due to congestion of pelvic vasculature.

TABLE 3-1. **Fundal Height During Pregnancy**

WEEKS PREGNANT	FUNDAL HEIGHT
12	Barely palpable above pubic symphysis
15	Midpoint between pubic symphysis and umbilicus
20	At the umbilicus
28	6 cm above the umbilicus
32	6 cm below the xyphoid process
36	2 cm below xyphoid process
40	4 cm below xiphoid process[a]

[a] Due to engagement and descent of the fetal head, the fundal height at 40 weeks is typically less than the fundal height at 36 weeks.

HOW?

The beta subunit of human chorionic gonadotropin (hCG) is detected in maternal serum or urine.

- hCG is a glycoprotein produced by the developing placenta shortly after implantation.
- A monoclonal antibody to the hCG antigen is utilized; the hCG–antibody complex is measured qualitatively.

Pregnancy tests not only detect hCG produced by the syncytiotrophoblast cells in the placenta, but also in:

- Hydatidiform mole
- Choriocarcioma
- Other germ cell tumors
- Ectopically producing breast cancers and large cell carcinoma of the lung

WHEN?

- Blood levels become detectably elevated 8–10 days after fertilization (3–3.5 weeks after the LMP).
- hCG rises in a geometric fashion during the first trimester, producing different ranges for each week of gestation:

Duration of Pregnancy (from Time of Ovulation)	Plasma hCG (mU/mL)
1 week	5–50
2 weeks	50–500
3 weeks	100–10,000
4 weeks	1,000–30,000
5 weeks	3,500–115,000
6–8 weeks	12,000–270,000
8–12 weeks	15,000–220,000
20–40 weeks	3,000–15,000

Urine hCG

- Preferred method to recognize normal pregnancy.
- Total urine hCG closely parallels plasma concentration.
- First morning specimens have less variability in relative concentration and generally higher levels, improving accuracy.
- Assays detecting 25 mU/mL recognize pregnancy with 95% sensitivity by 1 week after the first missed menstrual period.
- False negatives may occur if:
  - The test is performed too early.
  - The urine is very dilute.
- False positives may occur with:
  - Proteinuria (confirm with plasma hCG).
  - Urinary tract infection (UTI).

hCG is a glycoprotein hormone composed of alpha and beta subunits.

hCG is similar in structure and function to luteinizing hormone (the beta subunits are similar in both hormones).

The hCG alpha subunit is identical to that in luteinizing hormone (LH), follicle-stimulating hormone (FSH), and thyroid-stimulating hormone (TSH).

Plasma hCG levels should increase by 66–100% every 48 hours prior to 9–10 weeks.

HIGH-YIELD FACTS

Diagnosis of Pregnancy

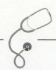

Serial hCGs are used to follow and make prognosis of first-trimester bleeding.

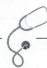

Do not assay for hCG before a woman has missed a menstrual period because of low test sensitivity before this time.

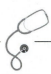

If FHTs are not auscultated by 11 weeks' GA, an ultrasonic evaluation should be performed to document a viable intrauterine pregnancy.

Scan dating is useful up to 20 weeks' GA when menstrual data is unreliable or conflicts with clinical findings.

Plasma hCG

Used when quantitative information is needed:
- To aid in diagnosing ectopic pregnancy
- Monitoring trophoblastic tumors
- Screening for fetal abnormalities
- Serial levels checked to rule out spontaneous abortion (< 10 weeks)

Do not provide cost-effective additional information in diagnosing routine pregnancy since they are positive < 1 week before urine hCG.

FETAL HEART TONES (FHTs)

The electronic Doppler device can detect fetal heart tones as early as 8 weeks' GA, albeit with difficulty.

ULTRASONIC SCANNING (US)

Not generally used to diagnose pregnancy, but can do so once a gestation sac is present within the uterus.

WHEN?

- To confirm an intrauterine pregnancy (if it is suspected to be ectopic).
- To confirm the presence of a fetal heartbeat in a patient with a history of miscarriage.
- To diagnose multiple pregnancy.
- To estimate gestational age.
- To screen for fetal structural anomalies.

Limitations

Scan dating becomes progressively less accurate after 20 weeks' GA. It can be used later, keeping in mind its limitations.
- US measures the size of the fetus, not the gestational age.
- Biologic variation in size increases as gestation advances.

Physiology of Pregnancy

General Effects of Pregnancy on the Mother   24

Normal Anatomical Adaptations in Pregnancy   35

Conception   36

Pregnancy Proteins   39

Pregnancy Steroids   39

First trimester (T1): 1–12 weeks

Second trimester (T2): 13–28 weeks

Third trimester (T3): 28 weeks–term

Term: 38–42 weeks

Joint changes (i.e., pubic symphysis) + postural changes secondary to change in center of gravity result in backaches and other aches that are common in pregnancy.

If normal prepregnancy weight: Patient should gain 25 to 35 lb during pregnancy. There should be little weight gain in T1, with most of weight gain in T2 and T3.

Ideal weight gain:
T1: 1.5–3 lb gained
T2 and T3: 0.8 lb/wk

Table 4-1 summarizes maternal physiologic changes during pregnancy.

Total Body Water

Increased by an average of 8.5 L and is composed of:

- Fetal water
- Amniotic fluid
- Placental tissue
- Maternal tissue
- Edema
- Generalized swelling leading to corneal swelling, intraocular pressure changes, gingival edema, increased vascularity of cranial sinuses, tracheal edema
- Increased hydration of connective tissue ground substance, leading to laxity and swelling of connective tissue and changes in joints that mainly occur in T3

Energy Requirements

Energy requirements increase gradually from 10 weeks to 36 weeks by 50–100 kcal/day. In the final 4 weeks, requirements increase by 300 kcal/day.

Metabolism

- Metabolic modifications begin soon after conception and are most marked in the second half of pregnancy, when fetal growth requirements increase.
- The uterus and placenta require carbohydrates, fats, and amino acids.

CARBOHYDRATE

The placenta is freely permeable to glucose, which increases availability to the fetus.

First 20 Weeks

Insulin sensitivity increases in first half of pregnancy.
- Fasting glucose levels are lower.
- This favors glycogen synthesis and storage, fat deposition, and amino acid transport into cells.

After 20 Weeks

Insulin resistance develops and plasma insulin levels rise.
- A carbohydrate load produces a rise in plasma insulin 3–4 times greater than in the nonpregnant state, but glucose levels also are higher.
- This reduces maternal utilization of glucose and induces glycogenolysis, gluconeogenesis, and maternal utilization of lipids as energy source.
- Despite these high and prolonged rises in postprandial plasma glucose, the fasting level in late pregnancy remains less than nonpregnant levels.

TABLE 4-1. Summary of Changes in the Body During Pregnancy

	FIRST TRIMESTER	SECOND TRIMESTER	THIRD TRIMESTER	DURING LABOR	9-MONTH PERIOD
Body water					↑ by 8.5 L
Energy requirements		↑ by 50–100 kcal/d	↑ by 300 kcal/d		
Body weight	↑ (primarily reflects maternal growth)	↑ (primarily reflects maternal growth)	↑ (primarily reflects fetal growth)		↑ by 25–35 lb
Tidal volume	↑				↑ by 200 mL
Vital capacity	↑				↑ by 100–200 mL
Cardiac output (CO)	↑ by 60%			↑ by 30% during each contraction May ↑ further in second stage of labor	↑
Blood pressure (BP)		↓		↑ by 10–20 mm Hg during each contraction May ↑ further in second stage of labor	
Systolic BP	↔				
Diastolic BP	↓	↓ by 15 mm Hg at 16–20 wks	↑ to T1 level		
Heart rate (HR)	↑ by 10–15%/min			↔	
Stroke volume (SV)	↑ by 10%			↑ During each contraction	
Central venous pressure	↔			↑ of 3–5 mm Hg during each contraction	
Systemic vascular resistance	↓ from pre-pregnancy level	↓↓ from pre-pregnancy level	↑, but not to prepregnancy level	↑ with each contraction	
Glomerular filtration rate (GFR)	↑	↑ to 60% above nonpregnant levels by 16 wks			↑

TABLE 4-1. Summary of Changes in the Body During Pregnancy (continued)

HIGH-YIELD FACTS

Physiology of Pregnancy

	FIRST TRIMESTER	SECOND TRIMESTER	THIRD TRIMESTER	DURING LABOR	9-MONTH PERIOD
Renal plasma flow	↑	↑ to 30–50% above nonpregnant levels by 20 wks	Peaks at 30 wks		↑
Plasma aldosterone	↑ w/in 2 wks of conception	↑ 3–5 times the nonpregnant level	↑ 8–10 times the nonpregnant level		↑
Serum alkaline phosphatase					↑
Plasma prolactin	↑				↑ 10–20 times nonpregnant level
Cortisol and other corticosteroids	↑ from 12 wks	↑	↑		↑ to 3–5 times nonpregnant levels
Glucagon					↑
Insulin sensitivity	↑	↓ at 20 wks	↓		
Fasting insulin levels		↑ at 20 wks	Peak at 32 wks		
Plasma volume	↑	↑	↑		↑ by 50%
Red blood cell (RBC) mass	↑	↑	↑		↑ by 18–30%
Mean corpuscular volume (MCV)	↔ or ↑ from 82–84 fL		↑ from 86–100 fL or more		
Neutrophils	↑	↑	↑ to 30 wks		
Erythrocyte sedimentation rate (ESR)	↑				↑
Albumin blood levels	↓	↓ from 3.5–2.5 g/100 mL	↓ by 22%		
Total globulin		↑ by 0.2 g/100 mL			
Total proteins		↓ by 20 wks from 7–6 g/100 mL			

TABLE 4-1. Summary of Changes in the Body During Pregnancy (continued)

	FIRST TRIMESTER	SECOND TRIMESTER	THIRD TRIMESTER	DURING LABOR	9-MONTH PERIOD
Thyroxine-binding globulin					↑ (Thyroxine-binding globulin levels double)
Total plasma cholesterol	↓ by 5%	↑	↑		↑ by 24–206%
Low-density lipoprotein (LDL)					↑ by 50–90%
Very low-density lipoprotein (VLDL)			Peaks at 36 wks		↑ by 36%
High-density lipoprotein (HDL)		↑ by 30%	Decreases from T2		↑ by 10–23%
Triglycerides			Reach 2–4 times nonpregnant level at 36 wks		↑ by 90–570%
Lipoprotein (a)	↑	↑ until 22 wks	↓ to nonpregnant levels		↔
Uterine contractions		Begin at 20 wks	↑		

AMINO ACIDS

- Plasma concentration of amino acids falls during pregnancy due to hemodilution.
- Urea synthesis is reduced.

LIPIDS

- All lipid levels are raised, with the greatest increases being in the triglyceride-rich component.
- Lipids cross the placenta.
- Hyperlipidemia of pregnancy is *not* atherogenic, but may unmask a pathologic hyperlipidemia.

Fat
- Early in pregnancy, fat is deposited.
- By midpregnancy, fat is the primary source of maternal energy.
- Postpartum, lipid levels return to normal (may take 6 months).

Cholesterol
- There is an increased turnover of cholesterol from lipoproteins, creating an increased supply to most tissues and increased supply for steroid production.

Goal in pregnancy is to increase the availability of glucose for the fetus, while the mother utilizes lipids.

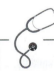

The optimal time to screen for glucose intolerance is at 26 to 28 weeks' GA.

- Total cholesterol is raised postpartum in all mothers, but can be reduced by dieting after delivery.

Triglycerides, very-low-density lipoprotein (VLDL), low-density lipoprotein (LDL), and high-density lipoprotein (HDL) increase during pregnancy.

DRUGS/OTHER SUBSTANCES

- Plasma levels of phenytoin fall during pregnancy.
- The half-life of caffeine is doubled.
- Antibiotics are cleared more rapidly by the kidney.

Central Nervous System

Syncope may occur from multiple etiologies:

1. Venous pooling in lower extremities leading to dizziness/light-headedness, especially with abrupt positional changes
2. Dehydration
3. Hypoglycemia
4. Postprandial shunting of blood flow to the stomach
5. Overexertion during exercise

Emotional and psychiatric symptoms may result from:
- Hormonal changes of pregnancy
- Progesterone (fatigue, dyspnea, depression)
- Endogenous corticosteroids (euphoria)

Respiratory System

Fetal P_{CO_2} must be greater than maternal P_{CO_2}; thus, the maternal respiratory center must be reset. This is done in several ways:
- During pregnancy, progesterone reduces the carbon dioxide threshold at which the respiratory center is stimulated and increases the respiratory center sensitivity. This may lead to hyperventilation of pregnancy.
- Tidal volume (TV) increases by 200 mL.
- Vital capacity (VC) increases by 100–200 mL.

Cardiovascular System

CARDIAC OUTPUT

- Cardiac output (CO) increases by 40% by week 10, due to a 10% increase in stroke volume (SV) and increase in heart rate (HR) by 10–15% per minute.
- Generalized enlargement of the heart and enlargement of left ventricle.
- Heart is displaced anterolaterally secondary to rise in level of diaphragm, which leads to altered electrocardiogram (ECG) and possible changes that mimic ischemia.
- **T1 and T2:** Decrease in BP secondary to decreased peripheral vascular resistance.

Physical Exam
- At end of T1—both components of S_1 become louder, with exaggerated splitting.

Normal pregnancy state is:
- Hyperlipemic
- Glycosuric
- Anabolic

The increase in cholesterol excretion results in increased risk of gallstones.

Healthy women must be treated as potential cardiac patients during pregnancy and the puerperium until functional murmurs resolve and the cardiovascular system returns to baseline status.

- After midpregnancy—90% of pregnant women demonstrate a third heart sound or S₃ gallop.
- **Systolic ejection murmurs** along the left sternal border occur in 96% of pregnant patients (due to increased flow across aortic and pulmonic valves).
- **Diastolic murmurs** are *never normal*, and their presence warrants evaluation by a cardiologist.

During Labor
- CO increases by 30% during each contraction due to an increase in SV, but no increase in HR.

VENOUS SYSTEM

Venous dilation results from:
- Relaxation of vascular smooth muscle.
- Pressure of enlarging uterus on inferior vena cava and iliac veins.

Gastrointestinal System

Reflux esophagitis (heartburn):
- Enlarging uterus displaces the stomach above the esophageal sphincter and causes increased intragastric pressure.
- Progesterone causes a relative relaxation of the esophageal sphincter.
- There may also be reflux of bile into the stomach due to pyloric incompetence.
- **Constipation** may occur secondary to progesterone, which relaxes intestinal smooth muscle and slows peristalsis.

GALLBLADDER
- Increases in size
- Empties more slowly
- **Cholestasis,** probably due to a hormonal effect since it also occurs in some users of oral contraceptives (OCs) and hormone replacement therapy (HRT)

LIVER
- Hepatic function increases.
- Plasma globulin and fibrinogen concentrations increase.
- Synthetic rate of albumin increases → total albumin mass increases by 19%, plateaus at 28 weeks.
- Velocity of blood flow in hepatic veins decreases.
- Serum alkaline phosphatase increases largely due to placental production.

Genitourinary System
- **Urinary stasis** secondary to decreased ureteral peristalsis and mechanical compression of the ureter (by the uterus) at pelvic brim as pregnancy progresses.
- **Asymptomatic bacteriuria** occurs in 5–8% of pregnant women (should be treated).

Patients with hypertensive heart disease may develop progressive or sudden deterioration (cardiomyopathy of pregnancy).

Increased distensibility and pressure of veins → predisposition to development of varicose veins of legs, vulva, rectum, and pelvis.

Decreased GI motility may be responsible for the increased absorption of water, Na⁺, and other substances.

The superior rectal vein is part of the portal system and has no valves, hence the high pressure within the system is communicated to the pelvic veins and produces **hemorrhoids.**

Cholestasis plus increase in lipids and cholesterol lead to higher incidence of gallstones, cholecystitis, and biliary obstruction.

- **Urinary frequency increases:**
  - During first 3 months of pregnancy due to bladder compression by enlarging uterus.
  - During last week of pregnancy as the fetal head descends into pelvis.
- **Nocturia:**
  - Physiologic after T1.
  - Passing urine up to four times per night is normal.
  - Fetal movements and insomnia contribute to the nocturia.
- **Stress incontinence:**
  - Occurs frequently during normal pregnancy.
  - Due to relaxation of the bladder supports.
  - The urethra normally elongates during pregnancy, but not in those who develop stress incontinence.

BLADDER

Bladder tone decreases, but bladder capacity increases progressively during pregnancy.

URETERS

Ureters undergo progressive dilatation and kinking in > 90% of pregnant women at ≥ 6 weeks.
- Accompanied by a decreased urine flow rate.
- Dilatation is greater on right secondary to dextrorotation of the uterus, and does not extend below the pelvic brim.
- Dilatation is secondary to the physical obstruction by the pregnant uterus and the effects of pregnancy hormones.
- Ureteric dilatation extends up to the calyces, leading to increased glomerular size and increased interstitial fluid, which causes enlarged kidneys (length increases by 1 cm and weight increases by 20%).

RENAL FUNCTION

- Renal plasma flow increases from T1, reaching 30–50% above nonpregnant levels by 20 weeks. Flow remains elevated until 30 weeks and then slowly declines to nonpregnant levels postpartum.
- Glomerular filtration rate (GFR) increases soon after conception. It reaches 60% above nonpregnant level by 16 weeks and remains elevated for remainder of pregnancy.

RENAL TUBULE CHANGES

Tubular function changes:
- Tubules lose some of their resorptive capacity—amino acids, uric acid, and glucose are not as completely absorbed in the pregnant female.
- Results in an increase in protein loss of up to 300 mg/24 hr.

Renal retention of Na+ results in water retention. Mother and conceptus increase their Na+ content by 500–900 nmol (due to increased reabsorption by renal tubules).

Albumin concentration falls by 22% due to hemodilution, despite the increase in synthetic rate.

Bacteruria + urinary stasis predispose patients to pyelonephritis, the most common nonobstetric cause for hospitalization during pregnancy.

In pregnancy, the increased rate of renal clearance leads to reduced effective dose of antibiotics and other medications.

Hematologic

PLASMA VOLUME

Plasma volume increases by 50% during pregnancy due to increase in both red blood cells (RBCs) and plasma, but proportionately more plasma. This results in hemodilution.

- Greater in multigravidas than primigravidas.
- Greater in multiple pregnancies than in single pregnancies.
- Positively correlated with birth weight.
- Increase in plasma volume is less in patients with recurrent abortions.
- Advantage of increased circulating volume:
    - Helps to compensate for increased blood flow to uterus and kidneys.
    - Reduces viscosity of blood and increases capillary blood flow.

RED BLOOD CELLS

- Circulating RBC mass increases progressively during pregnancy:
    - By 18% in women not given Fe supplements.
    - By 30% in women on Fe supplementation.
- Reticulocyte count increases by $\geq 2\%$.
- Mean corpuscular volume (MCV) usually increases.

HEMOGLOBIN

Fetal Hgb (HbF) concentration increases 1–2% during pregnancy, secondary to an increase in the number of RBCs with HbF.

ERYTHROCYTE SEDIMENTATION RATE (ESR)

- Rises early in pregnancy due to the increase in fibrinogen and other physiologic changes.
- An ESR = 100 mm/hr is not uncommon in normal pregnancy.

WHITE BLOOD CELLS

Neutrophils
- Neutrophil count increases in T1 and continues to rise until 30 weeks.
- Neutrophilic metabolic activity and phagocytic function increases.

Lymphocytes
- Counts remain unchanged, but function is suppressed.

PLATELETS

- Platelet reactivity is increased in T2 and T3 and returns to normal at 12 weeks postpartum.
- In 8–10% of normal pregnancies, the platelet count falls below 150×10^3 without negative effects on the fetus.

COAGULATION

- Pregnancy is a hypercoagulable state (risk factor for stroke, pulmonary emboli, deep venous thrombosis).
- Hypercoagulable disorders may become apparent during pregnancy.

GFR increases; quantity of glucose filtered in urine is greater than in nonpregnant state; tubular threshold for glucose is variable. Glycosuria is detected in 50% of pregnant women.

Tubules are presented with increased quantities of urine because of the increased GFR.

Progesterone increases Na^+ excretion, but its increase is balanced by effects of increased aldosterone, mineralocorticoids, and prostaglandins.

Endocrine System

In general, the endocrine system is modified in the pregnancy state by the addition of the fetoplacental unit. The fetoplacental unit produces human chorionic gonadotropin (hCG) and human placental lactogen (hPL), among other hormones.

- **hCG** (luteotropic): Coregulates and stimulates adrenal and placental steroidogenesis. Stimulates fetal testes to secrete testerone. Possesses thyrotrophic activity.
- **hPL** (also called human chorionic somatomammotropin [hCS]): Anti-insulin and growth hormone–like effects lead to impaired maternal glucose and free fatty acid release.

PITUITARY GLAND

The pituitary gland increases in weight and sensitivity during pregnancy.

Prolactin
- Plasma levels rise within a few days postconception.
- At term, levels are 10- to 20-fold higher than nonpregnant state.

Follicle-Stimulating Hormone
- Blunted response to gonadotropin-releasing hormone (GnRH).
- Shows a progressive decreased response; no response at 3 weeks after ovulation.

Luteinizing Hormone
- Response to GnRH diminishes and finally disappears.

ADRENAL GLAND

- Plasma cortisol and other corticosteroids increase progressively from 12 weeks to term and reach 3–5 times nonpregnant levels.
- Half-life of plasma cortisol is increased, while its clearance is reduced.

THYROID GLAND

- Total thyroxine levels and thyroxine-binding globulin increase. The result is that *free thyroxine remains normal and the mother remains euthyroid.*
- The thyroid gland itself does not increase in size. All goiters should be investigated.

PARATHYROID GLANDS

- Calcitriol (1,25-dihydroxycholecalciferol) levels increase in pregnancy, which increases maternal calcium absorption, to offset maternal losses across the placenta to the fetus.
- At term, serum parathyroid hormone levels are higher in the mother, but calcitonin is higher in the fetus. This results in fetal bone deposition.
- Parathyroid hormone (PTH) concentration **falls.** PTH-related protein increases.

PLASMA PROTEINS

Concentrations of proteins in maternal serum *fall markedly by 20 weeks, mostly due to a fall in serum albumin.* This fall reduces the colloid osmotic pressure in the plasma → edema in pregnancy.

PANCREAS

- Size of islets of Langerhans increases during pregnancy.
- The number of beta cells increases during pregnancy.
- The number of insulin receptor sites increases during pregnancy.

Insulin

- Serum levels rise during second half of pregnancy, but insulin resistance increases as well.
- This insulin resistance may be due to presence of hPL, prolactin, or other pregnancy hormones that have anti-insulin activity.
- Insulin resistance switches carbohydrate to fat utilization.

Glucagon

- Levels are slightly raised in pregnancy, but not as much as insulin levels.

Integumentary System/Skin

Many physiologic changes in the skin can occur during gestation. Some are believed to result from changes in the hormonal milieu of pregnancy (see Table 4-2).

MELANOCYTE-STIMULATING HORMONE EFFECTS

Melanocyte-stimulating hormone increases can result in the following:
- **Linea nigra:** Black line/discoloration of the abdomen that runs from above the umbilicus to the pubis; may be seen during the latter part of gestation.
- **Darkening of nipple and areola.**
- **Facial chloasma/melasma:** A light- or dark-brown hyperpigmentation in exposed areas such as the face. More common in persons with brown or black skin color, who live in sunny areas, and who are taking OCs.
- A suntan acquired in pregnancy lasts longer than usual.

ESTROGEN EFFECTS

- Spider nevi are common (branched growths of dilated capillaries on the skin).
- Palmar erythema.

CORTICOSTEROID EFFECTS

Striae on the abdomen, breasts, etc., develop in response to increased circulating corticosteroids. Other factors lead to a decrease in elastin and fibrillin and mechanical stretching.

FINGERNAILS

Grow more rapidly during pregnancy.

Pregnancy and combinations of estrogen and progestational agents (i.e., OCs and HRT) are the most frequent causes of melasma (often called the **"mask of pregnancy"**).

TABLE 4-2. Pruritic Dermatologic Disorders Unique to Pregnancy

DISEASE	ONSET	PRURITIS	LESIONS	DISTRIBUTION	INCIDENCE	INCREASED INCIDENCE FETAL MORBIDITY/ MORTALITY	INTERVENTION
Pruritic urticarial papules and plaques of pregnancy (PUPPP) (polymorphic eruption of pregnancy)	T2–T3	Severe	Erythematous urticarial papules and plaques	Abdomen, thighs, buttocks, occasionally arms and legs	Common (1:160– 1:300)	No	Topical steroids, antipruritic drugs (hydroxy-zine, diphenhy-dramine)
Papular eruptions (prurigo gestationis and papular dermatitis)	T2–T3	Severe	Excoriated papules	No area of predilection	Uncommon (1:300– 1:2,400)	Unlikely	Systemic/ topical cortico-steroids, an-tipruritics
Pruritus gravidarum	T3	Severe	Excoriations common	Generalized	Common (1–2%)	Yes	Antipruritics, cholestyra-mine
Impetigo herpetiformis (pustular psoriasis of pregnancy)	T3	Minimal	Pustules	Genitalia, medial thighs, umbilicus, breasts, axillae	Rare	Yes (maternal sepsis common)	Systemic cortico-steroids and antibiotics for sec-ondary infection
Herpes gestationis (pemphigoid gestationis)	T2– post-partum	Severe	Erythematous papules, vesicles, bullae	Abdomen, extremities, generalized	Rare (1:1,700– 50,000)	Yes (growth restriction and pre-maturity)	*Mild*—topical steroids, antihista-mines *More severe*— systemic cortico-steroids

PTH and calcitonin do *not* cross the placenta.

HAIR

- The rate at which hair is shed is reduced.
- The excess retained hair is often lost in the puerperium.

Vagina

- Vaginal epithelium hypertrophies and quantity of glycogen-containing cells shed into vagina increase.
- Connective tissue decreases in collagen content and there is an increase in water content (like the cervix—*see below*).
- Vagina becomes more acidic (pH = 4–5), which hinders growth of most pathogens and favors growth of yeasts.

Uterus

- Hypertrophy and hyperplasia of myometrial smooth muscle (which contains estrogen and progesterone receptors) secondary to:
  - Action of steroid hormones.
  - Uterine distention and wall thinning with the growing fetus, placenta, amniotic fluid.
- Term uterus weighs 1,100 g with a 20-fold increase in mass (nonpregnant, parous uterus weighs 70 g).

ROUND LIGAMENT

Round ligament increases in length, muscular content, and diameter:
- During pregnancy, the ligaments may contract spontaneously or in response to uterine movement.
- In labor, contractions of the ligaments pull the uterus forward, which leads to expulsive force directed as much into the pelvis as possible.

VASCULAR SUPPLY OF THE UTERUS

- In the nonpregnant state, the uterine artery is most important blood source.
- During pregnancy, the ovarian arteries contribute 20–30% of the blood supply in 70% of women.
- Uterine arteries dilate to 1.5 times their nonpregnant diameter.

UTERINE CERVIX

The amount of collagen within the cervix is reduced to one third of the nonpregnant amount. The duration of spontaneous labor is inversely proportional to cervical collagen concentration at the beginning of dilation.

Accumulation of glycosaminoglycans and increase in water content and vascularity in the cervix results in **softening** and cyanosis = characteristic cervix of gravid female:
- Results in increased compliance to stretch.
- This process is called "**cervical ripening**" and takes place gradually over the last few weeks of gestation.
- In early T1, squamous epithelium of ectocervix becomes hyperactive, endocervical glands become hyperplastic, and endocervical epithelium proliferates and grows out over the ectocervix.
- The resulting secretions within the endocervical canal create the **antibacterial mucous plug of the cervix.**
- Cervical effacement causes expulsion of the mucous plug as the cervical canal is shortened during labor.

- The uterine isthmus is normally a small region of the uterus that lies between the uterine corpus and cervix.
- Beginning at 12 weeks of pregnancy, the isthmus enlarges and thins secondary to hormonal influences of pregnancy and uterine distention.
- During labor, the isthmus expands and is termed the *lower uterine segment*.

CONCEPTION

Ovulation

Ovulation is necessary for normal fertilization to occur:
- The ovum must leave the ovary and be carried into the fallopian tube.
- The unfertilized ovum is surrounded by its zona pellucida.
- This oocyte has completed its first meiotic division and carries its first polar body.

Fertilization

Fertilization typically occurs within 24 hours after ovulation in the third of the fallopian tube adjacent to the ovary (ampulla):
- The sperm penetrates the zona pellucida and fuses its plasma membranes with those of the ovum.
- The sperm nucleus and other cellular contents enter the egg's cytoplasm.
- Fertilization signals the ovum to complete meiosis II and to discharge an additional polar body.

Preimplantation

- The fertilized ovum remains in the ampulla for 80 hours after follicular rupture and travels through the isthmus of the fallopian tube for 10 hours.
- The fertilized egg divides to form a multicellular blastomere.
- The blastomere passes from the fallopian tube into the uterine cavity.
- The embryo develops into a **blastocyst** as it freely floats in endometrial cavity 90–150 hours after conception (see Table 4-3).

Implantation

- On day 5–6 of development, the blastocyst adheres to the endometrium with the help of adhesion molecules on the secretory endometrial surface.
- After attachment, the endometrium proliferates around the blastocyst.

Placentation

- During week 2, cells in the outer cell mass differentiate into **trophoblasts.**

TABLE 4-3. Embryology

Week	Preembryonic Period
1	Fertilization and start of implantation.
2	Formation of yolk sac and embryonic disk.
3	First missed menstrual period; formation of primitive streak and neural groove.

Embryonic Period

4	Primitive heartbeat; crown–rump length (CRL) approximately 4.0 mm.
5	Hand and foot plates develop.
6	Hand plates develop digital rays; upper lip, nose, and external ear formed.
7	Umbilical herniation (intestines begin growth outside abdominal cavity).
8	Human appearance; tail has disappeared; CRL approximately 30 mm.

Previable Fetal Period

9	Eyes closing or closed.
10	Intestines in abdomen; thyroid, pancreas, and gallbladder development.
11	Fetal kidneys begin excreting urine into amniotic fluid; fetal liver begins to function; baby teeth formed in sockets.
12	Sex distinguishable externally; fetal breathing movements begin; colonic rotation; fetus active; first-trimester ends.
14	Head and neck take an erect, straight-line alignment.
16	Increased fetal activity; ultrasound can determine sex; myelination of nerves and ossification of bones begins.
18	Egg cells, ovaries, and uterus develop in females.
20	Head and body (lanugo) visible; testes begin descent in males.

Viable Fetal Period

22	Fetus can hear, will reflexively move in response to loud noise.
26	Fetal lungs develop alveoli and secrete surfactant, fetus generally capable of breathing air by week 27.
28	Third trimester begins; eyelids unfuse; muscle tone increases.
30	Cerebral gyri and sulci, which began to form in week 26, are now prominent and begin accelerated formation.

Human chorionic gonadotropin (hCG) is detectable in maternal serum after implantation has taken place, approximately 8 to 11 days after conception.

Trophoblasts (trophoectoderm) are the precursor cells for the placenta and membranes.

HIGH-YIELD FACTS

Physiology of Pregnancy

TABLE 4-3. Embryology (continued)

Week	Preembryonic Period
32	Fetal immune system functioning and capable of responding to mild infections.
34	Vernix thickens.
36	Fetus capable of sucking; meconium present in fetal intestines.
38	Fetus described as "full-term" at this point.
40	Due date.

- A trophoblastic shell forms the initial boundary between the embryo and the endometrium.
- The trophoblasts nearest the myometrium form the placental disk; the other trophoblasts form the chorionic membranes.

Postimplantation

- The endometrium or lining of the uterus during pregnancy is termed *decidua*.
- Maternal RBCs may be seen in the trophoblastic lacunae in the second week postconception.

The decidua produces maternal steroids and synthesizes proteins that are related to the maintenance and protection of the pregnancy from immunologic rejection.

The Placenta

The placenta continues to adapt over T2 and T3. It is the **primary producer of steroid hormones** after 7 weeks' gestational age.

Blood Supply

Flow in the arcuate and radial arteries during normal pregnancy is high with low resistance (resistance falls after 20 weeks).

Developmental Ages

Postconception Day	Tissue/Organ Formation
4	Blastula
7–12	Implantation
13	Primitive streak
16	Neural plate
19–21	First somite
23–25	Closure of anterior neuropore
25–27	Arms bud
	Closure of posterior neuropore
28	Legs bud
44	Sexual differentiation

38

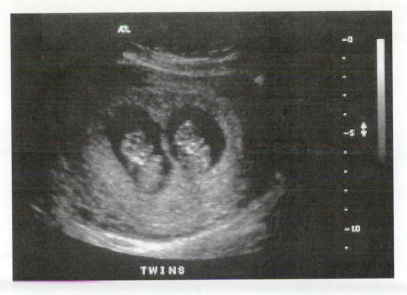

FIGURE 4-1. US of dizygotic twins.

(Courtesy of Dr. James and Mrs. Kirstin Homme.)

Multiple Gestation (Figure 4-1)

- Division of embryos before differentiation of trophoblast (between days 2 and 3) → two chorions, two amnions.
- Division of embryos after trophoblast differentiation and before amnion formation (between days 3 and 8) → one placenta, one chorion, two amnions.
- Division of embryos after amnion formation (between days 8 and 13) → one placenta, one chorion, one amnion.
- Later division (> 13 d) conjoined twins.

PREGNANCY PROTEINS

Table 4-4 lists pregnancy proteins.

PREGNANCY STEROIDS

Estrogens affect uterine vasculature, placental steroidogenesis, and parturition. (See Figure 4-2.) Table 4-5 lists pregnancy steroids.

TABLE 4-4. Pregnancy Proteins

PROTEIN	SOURCE	FUNCTION
hCG	Placenta	Maintains the corpus luteum. Stimulates adrenal and placental steroido-genesis.
ACTH	Trophoblasts	Stimulates an increase in circulating maternal free cortisol.
hPL	Trophoblasts	Antagonizes insulin → maternal glucose intolerance, lipolysis, and proteolysis.
CRH	Placental tissue, decidua, hypo-thalamus (maternal)	Stimulates placental ACTH release and participates in the surge of fetal gluco-corticoids associated with late T3 fetal maturation. Cortisol has feedback with placental CRH production.
Prolactin	Decidualized endo-metrium	Regulates fluid and electrolyte flux through the fetal membranes.
AFP	Yolk sac, fetal gastro-intestinal tract, fetal liver	Regulates fetal intravascular volume (osmo-regulator). ■ Maternal AFP peaks between 10 and 13 weeks gestational age, then declines thereafter. ■ Detectable as early as 7 weeks' gestation.

ACTH, adrenocorticotropic hormone; AFP, alpha-fetoprotein; CRH, corticotropin-releasing hormone; hCG, human chorionic gonadotropin; hPL, human placental lactogen.

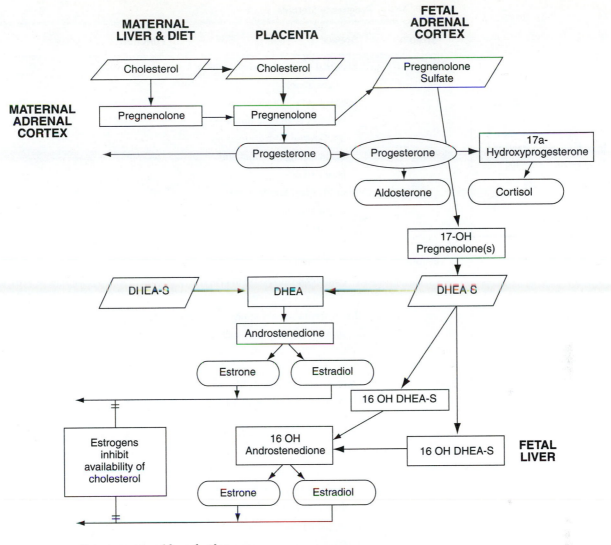

FIGURE 4-2. **Pregnancy steroid production.**

DHEA, dehydroepiandrosterone; DHEA-S, dehydroepiandrosterone sulfate, 16 OH DHEA-S, 16a-hydroxydehydroepiandrosterone sulfate.

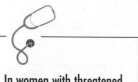

In women with threatened T1 abortions, estradiol concentrations are abnormally low for gestational age.

TABLE 4-5. Pregnancy Steroids

STEROID	SOURCE	FUNCTION
Estradiol	Maternal ovaries for weeks 1–6 of gestation. Subsequently, the placenta secretes increasing quantities synthesized from conversion of circulating maternal and fetal DHEA-S. After T1, the placenta is the major source of circulating estradiol.	
Estrone	Maternal ovaries, adrenals, and peripheral conversion in first 4–6 wks of pregnancy. The placenta subsequently secretes increasing quantities.	
Estriol	Placenta. Continued production is dependent on the presence of a living fetus.	
Progesterone	Corpus luteum before 6 weeks' gestational age. Thereafter, the placenta produces progesterone from circulating maternal LDL cholesterol.	Affects tubal motility, the endometrium, uterine vasculature, and parturition. Inhibits T lymphocyte–mediated tissue rejection. Low levels in T1 associated with ectopic pregnancy and intrauterine fetal demise. High levels associated with hydatidiform mole.
Cortisol	Decidual tissue.	Suppresses maternal immune rejection response of the implanted conceptus.
LDL cholesterol	Fetal adrenal gland.	Principal regulatory precursor of corpus luteum progesterone production. Principal lipoprotein utilized in fetal adrenal steroidogenesis.

DHEA-S, dehydroepiandrosterone sulfate; LDL, low-density lipoprotein.

Antepartum

Prenatal Care   44

Assessment of Gestational Age   44

The Triple Screen: Maternal Serum Screening   46

Rh Incompatibility and Pregnancy   47

Fetal Imaging   48

Nutritional Needs of the Pregnant Woman   51

Answers to Commonly Asked Questions   52

When to Call the Physician   56

Gravidity: The number of times a woman has been pregnant.
Parity: The number of times a woman has had a pregnancy that led to a birth after 20 weeks' gestation or an infant > 500 g.

PRENATAL CARE

Goal

To increase the probability of a healthy baby without maternal compromise.

When and How Often

- < 28 weeks: Every month
- 28 to 36 weeks: Every 2–3 weeks
- 36 weeks to delivery: Once per week until delivery

See Table 5-1.

Terminology of Reproductive History

The mother's pregnancy history is described in terms of gravidity (G) and parity (P), in which parity includes term births, preterm births, abortions, and living children. The order expressed is as follows: total number of times pregnant (gravidity); term births; preterm births; abortuses; living children.

The terminology is written as in the following example: **G3P1201.**

The above indicates that a woman has been pregnant three times, has had one term birth, two preterm births, no abortions, and has one live child.

Important Hallmarks in Prenatal Visits

First Visit
- Pap smear
- Rh screen
- STD screen
- Labs

Weeks 16–18
- First sonogram
- Amniocentesis (if indicated)
- Triple screen

Weeks 26–28
- Diabetes screen, CBC, RhoGAM—negative blood type

Week 36
- Group B strep culture

ASSESSMENT OF GESTATIONAL AGE

Definitions

Gestational age (GA): The time of pregnancy counting from the first day of the last menstrual period.
Developmental age: The time of pregnancy counting from fertilization
First trimester: 0–14 weeks
Second trimester: 14–28 weeks
Third trimester: 28 weeks–birth

TABLE 5-1. Prenatal Visits

FIRST VISIT	6–8 WEEKS	16–18 WEEKS	26–28 WEEKS
1. History and physical (H&P)	1. H&P	1. H&P	1. H&P
2. Labs:	2. Fetal exam:	2. Fetal exam:	2. Fetal exam:
■ Hct/Hgb	■ **Fetal heart tones**	■ Fetal heart	■ Fetal heart
■ Rh factor	3. Urine analysis and culture	■ Fundal height	■ Fundal height
■ Blood type	4. HIV testing (if repeat is warranted)	3. **Pelvic sonogram (optional)**	■ Fetal position
■ Antibody screen		4. Amniocentesis (if indicated)	3. Labs:
■ Pap smear		5. **Triple screen (serum alpha-fetoprotein, estriol, beta-hCG)**	■ Complete blood count
■ *Gonorrhea* and *Chlamydia* cultures		6. Urine analysis and culture	■ Ab screen
■ Urine analysis (glucose, proteins, ketones) and culture, microscopic exam for sediment			■ *Gonorrhea* and *Chlamydia* cultures (optional)
■ Infection screen: Rubella, syphilis, hepatitis B, human immunodeficiency virus (HIV), tuberculosis (TB)			■ **Diabetes screen**
3. Genetic screen			■ Urine analysis/culture
4. Patient education			■ Syphilis screen (optional)
			4. Give RhoGAM if nonsensitized Rh negative patient

WEEK 32	WEEK 36	WEEK 38	WEEK 39	WEEK 40
1. H&P	1. H&P	1. H&P	1. H&P	1. H&P
2. Fetal exam:	2. Fetal exam:	2. Fetal exam:	2. Fetal exam:	2. Fetal exam:
■ Fetal heart	■ Fetal heart	■ Fetal heart	■ Fetal heart	■ Fetal heart
■ Fundal height	■ Fundal height	■ Fundal height	■ Fundal height	■ Fundal height
■ Fetal position	■ Fetal position	■ Fetal position	■ Fetal position	■ Fetal position
3. Urine analysis/ culture	3. Urine analysis/ culture	3. Urine analysis/ culture	3. Urine analysis/ culture	3. Urine analysis/ culture
	4. **Group B strep culture**	4. **Cervical exam (frequency is controversial)**		4. **Fetoplacental functional tests (if indicated)**

Embryo: Fertilization–8 weeks
Fetus: 8 weeks–birth
Previable: Before 24 weeks
Preterm: 24–37 weeks
Term: 37–42 weeks

Naegele's Rule

■ Naegele's rule is used to calculate the estimated date of confinement (i.e., due date) +/– 2 weeks.

Naegele's rule assumes two things:
1. A normal gestation is 280 days.
2. All patients have a 28-day menstrual cycle.

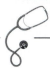

The first step in the workup of an abnormal triple screen should be an ultrasound for dating and anatomy.

Most NTDs are thought to be polygenic or multifactorial.

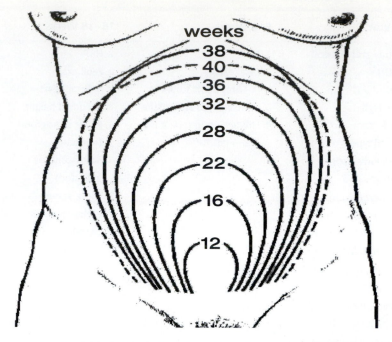

FIGURE 5-1. **Fundal height according to number of weeks of gestation.**

- First day of patient's last normal menstrual period − 3 months + 7 days + 1 year.
- Example: If LMP = July 20, 2006, then EDC = April 27, 2007.

Abdominal Exam and Fundal Height

As the fetus grows, the location of the uterus, or fundal height, grows superiorly in the abdomen, toward the maternal head. The location in the abdomen that the fetus and uterus are located is described in terms of weeks (see Figure 5-1).

- **Uterus at the level of umbilicus:** 20 weeks
- **Uterus at level of pubic symphysis:** 12 weeks
- **Uterus between pubic symphysis and umbilicus:** 16 weeks

THE TRIPLE SCREEN: MATERNAL SERUM SCREENING

Maternal Serum Alpha-Fetoprotein (MSAFP)

- Normally, MSAFP begins to rise at 13 weeks and peaks at 32 weeks. It is produced in the placenta.
- MSAFP screening is most accurate between 16 and 18 weeks.
- **An inaccurate gestational age is the most common reason for an abnormal screen.**

High levels are associated with:
- Neural tube defects (NTDs)
- Abdominal wall defects (gastroschisis and omphalocele)
- Fetal death

- Placental abnormalities (i.e., abruption)
- Multiple gestations

Low levels are associated with:
- Down syndrome (trisomy 21).
- One third to one fifth of Down syndrome fetuses exhibit low MSAFP.

Estriol

Low levels are associated with:
- **Trisomy 21** (Down syndrome)
- **Trisomy 18** (Edwards syndrome)
- Possibly low in **trisomy 13** (Patau syndrome)

Human Chorionic Gonadotropin (hCG)

High levels are associated with:
- Trisomy 21

Low levels are associated with:
- Trisomy 18
- Anencephaly

Rh INCOMPATIBILITY AND PREGNANCY

What Is Rh?

- The surface of the human red blood cell (RBC) may or may not contain a Rhesus (Rh) antigen. If so, that person is said to be Rhesus positive (for example, if someone with blood type A has a Rhesus antigen, the blood type is A+. If that person has no Rhesus antigen, he is A−).
- Half of all antigens in a fetus come from the father, and half come from the mother.

The Problem with Rh Sensitization

The parental combination you must worry about: mother Rh negative and father Rh positive.
- If the pregnant female is Rh negative and her fetus is Rh positive, then she may become sensitized to the Rh antigen and develop antibodies.
- These antibodies cross the placenta and attack the fetal RBCs, resulting in RBC hemolysis and erythroblastosis fetalis.

Sensitization

Sensitization may occur during:
- Amniocentesis
- Miscarriage/threatened abortion
- Vaginal bleeding
- Placental abruption/previa
- Delivery
- Abdominal trauma
- Cesarean section
- External version

Erythroblastosis fetalis

Hemolytic disease of the newborn/fetal hydrops occurs when the mother lacks an antigen present in the fetus → fetal RBCs trigger an immune response when they reach the mother's circulation → maternal antibodies cause fetal RBC hemolysis and anemia → fetal hyperbilirubinemia → kernicterus → heart failure, edema, ascites, pericardial effusion.

Suspected fetomaternal bleed—a **Kleihauer–Bettke** test is done to determine the amount of fetal RBCs in the maternal circulation. Adjustments in the amount of RhIgG are given to mother accordingly (see section on RhoGAM).

47

Scenario of Fetal Danger

Rh-negative mother becomes sensitized during an earlier pregnancy in which the child was Rh positive. She is exposed to Rh-positive blood during that pregnancy and/or delivery and develops antibodies. Then, in a later pregnancy, her immune system, already primed to recognize Rh-positive blood, crosses the placenta and attacks Rh-positive fetal blood.

Screening

In each pregnancy, a woman should have her Rh type determined and an antibody screen performed at the initial visit with an **indirect Coombs' test.**

RhoGAM: Treatment for Exposure

If the Rh-negative mother is exposed to fetal blood, **RhoGAM** is given. RhoGAM is Rh immune globulin (RhIgG—IgG that will attach to the Rh antigen and prevent immune response by the mother).

Management of the Unsensitized Rh-Negative Patient (The Rh-Negative Patient Who Has a Negative Antibody Screen)

1. Antibody screen should be done at 0, 24–28 weeks.
2. If negative, give 300 µg of RhIgG to prevent maternal development of antibodies.
3. At birth, determine if baby is Rh positive; if so, give postpartum RhIgG.

Management of the Sensitized Rh-Negative Patient (If on Initial Visit the Antibody Screen for Rh Is Positive)

1. Perform antibody screen at 0, 12–20 weeks.
2. Check the antibody titer.
   - If titer remains stable at < 1:16, the likelihood of hemolytic disease of the newborn is low.
   - If the titer is > 1:16 and/or rising, the likelihood of hemolytic disease of the newborn is high. Amniocentesis is done.
3. Amniocentesis begins at 16–20 weeks' GA.
   - Fetal cells are analyzed for Rh status.
   - Amniotic fluid is analyzed by spectrophotometer, which measures the light absorbance by bilirubin. Absorbance measurements can be graphically plotted to predict the severity of disease.
   - Serial US to rule out hydrops or IUGR.

FETAL IMAGING

Ultrasound

- Intrauterine pregnancy seen via vaginal ultrasound (US) when β-hCG is > 1,500.
- Intrauterine pregnancy seen via abdominal US when β-hCG is > 6,000.

- **Amniotic fluid index (AFI):** Represents the total of linear measurements (in centimeters) of the largest amniotic fluid pockets in each of the four quadrants of the amniotic fluid sac.
  - Reduced amniotic fluid volume (AFI < 5) = **oligohydramnios.**
  - Excessive fluid (AFI > 20) = **polyhydramnios.**
- See Figures 5-2 through 5-8 for normal and abnormal US findings.

Amniocentesis

Amniocentesis is the most extensively used fetal sampling technique and is typically performed at 15 weeks' GA, when the amniotic fluid is 200 mL.

Indications
- Fetal anomaly suspected on US.
- Abnormal MSAFP.
- Family history of congenital abnormalities.
- Offered to all patients ≥ 35 years of age.
- Assessment of fetal lung maturity.
- Others: Rule out infection, check hemoglobin, check bilirubin.

Procedure
- Thirty milliliters of amniotic fluid is removed via a 20- to 22-gauge needle using a transabdominal approach with US guidance.
- Biochemical analysis is performed on the extracted fluid:
  - Amniotic fluid AFP levels.
  - Fetal cells can be grown for karyotyping or DNA assays.

Risks
- Pain/cramping.
- Vaginal spotting (resolves spontaneously)/amniotic fluid leakage in 1–2% of cases.
- Symptomatic amnionitis in < 1/1,000 patients.
- **Rate of fetal loss is ≤ 0.5% (1/200) (less in experienced hands).**

Chorionic Villus Sampling (CVS)

Chorionic villus sampling is a diagnostic technique in which a small sample of chorionic villi is taken transcervically or transabdominally and analyzed.
- Typically done between 9 and 12 weeks' GA.
- Allows for chromosomal status, fetal karyotyping, and biochemical assays or DNA tests to be done earlier than amniocentesis.

Risks

- 0.5% rate of complications
  - Preterm delivery
  - Premature rupture of membranes
- Fetal injury

Cordocentesis

Cordocentesis is a procedure in which a spinal needle is advanced transabdominally under US guidance into a cord vessel to sample fetal blood. Typically performed after 17 weeks.

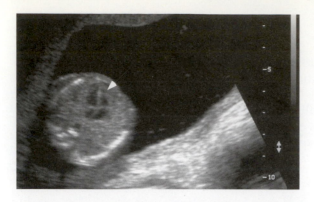

F I G U R E 5 - 2 . **Normal four-chamber heart.**

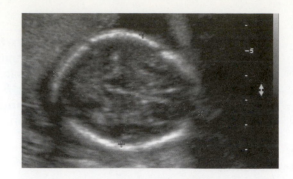

F I G U R E 5 - 3 . **Measurement of biparietal diameter.**

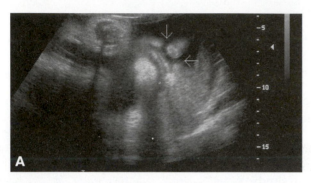

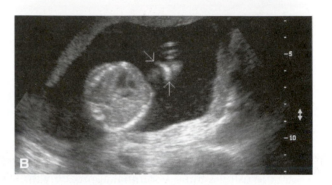

F I G U R E 5 - 4 . **A. Cleft lip (arrows).** **B. Normal lip (arrows).**

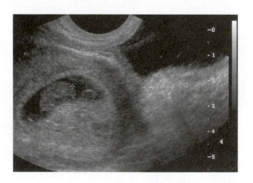

F I G U R E 5 - 5 . **Measurement of crown–rump length.**

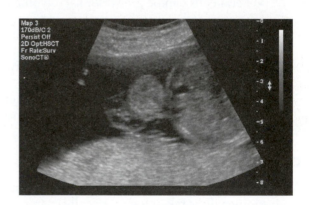

F I G U R E 5 - 6 . **Omphalocele.**

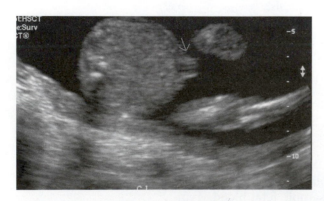

F I G U R E 5 - 7 . **Umbilical cord insertion.**

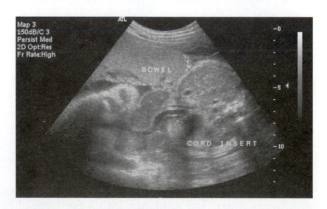

F I G U R E 5 - 8 . **Gastroschisis.**

Indications

- Fetal karyotyping because of fetal anomalies.
- To determine the fetal hematocrit in Rh isoimmunization or severe fetal anemia.
- To assay fetal platelet counts, acid–base status, antibody levels, blood chemistries, etc.

Genetic Testing

Genetic testing, if indicated, is performed with the following techniques:

- **FISH (fluorescent *in situ* hybridization):** A specific DNA probe with a fluorescent label that binds homologous DNA → allows identification of specific sites along a chromosome.
- **Karyotyping:** Allows visualization of chromosome size, banding pattern, and centromere position.

Indications

- Advanced maternal age
- Previous child with abnormal karyotype
- Parental chromosome rearrangements
- Fetal structural abnormality on sonogram
- Unexplained intrauterine growth retardation (IUGR)
- Abnormally low MSAFP

Polyhydramnios (AFI > 20) may signify poor control in a diabetic pregnancy, a fetal anomaly, multiple gestation, or infection.

NUTRITIONAL NEEDS OF THE PREGNANT WOMAN

Weight Gain

- Weight gain for normal BMI = **25–35 lb.**
- Optimal weight gain for an underweight teenager carrying a singleton pregnancy = 40 lb or 5 lb every 4 weeks in second half of pregnancy.
- An obese woman may need to gain only 15 lb.

Diet

The average woman must consume an additional **300 kcal/day** beyond baseline needs.

Vitamins

- **400 μg/day folic acid** is required. Ideal if started 3 months before pregnancy.
- **30 mg elemental iron per day is recommended in T2 and T3.** Total of 1 g iron is needed for pregnancy (500 mg for increase RBC mass, 300 mg for fetus, 200 mg for GI losses).
- The recommended dietary allowance (RDA) for calcium is increased in pregnancy to 1,200 mg/day and may be met adequately with diet alone.
- The RDA for zinc is increased from 15 to 20 mg/day.

BODY MASS INDEX (BMI)

$$BMI = \frac{weight\ (kg)}{height\ (m^2)}$$

BMI ≥ 30: Obese
25.0–29.9: Overweight
18.5–24.9: Normal
< 18.5: Underweight

Vegetarians

- *Lactoovovegetarians* in general have no nutritional deficiencies, except possibly iron and zinc.
- *Vegans* must consume sufficient quantities of vegetable proteins to provide all essential amino acids normally found in animal protein. Supplementation of zinc, vitamin B_{12}, and iron is necessary.

Pica

Occasionally seen in pregnancy, pica is the compulsive ingestion of nonfood substances with little or no nutritional value:

- Ice
- Clay (geophagia)
- Starch (amylophagia)

ANSWERS TO COMMONLY ASKED QUESTIONS

Caffeine in Pregnancy

- Contained in coffee, tea, chocolate, cola beverages.
- Ingestion of caffeine may increase risk of early spontaneous abortion among nonsmoking women carrying fetuses of normal karyotype. This risk increases according to amount of caffeine ingested (*NEJM* 2000;343:1839–1845).
- Adverse maternal effects include:
  - Insomnia
  - Acid indigestion
  - Reflux
  - Urinary frequency

Exercise

- No data exist to indicate that a pregnant woman must decrease the intensity of her exercise or lower her target heart rate.
- Women who exercised regularly before pregnancy should continue: Exercise may relieve stress, decrease anxiety, increase self-esteem, and shorten labor.
- The form of exercise should be one with low risk of trauma, particularly abdominal (water exercises are ideal).
- Exercise that requires prolonged time in the supine position should be avoided in T2 and T3.
- Exercise should be stopped if patient experiences oxygen deprivation (manifested by extreme fatigue, dizziness, or shortness of breath).
- Contraindications to exercise include:
  - Evidence of IUGR
  - Persistent vaginal bleeding
  - Incompetent cervix
  - Risk factors for preterm labor
  - Rupture of membranes
  - Pregnancy-induced hypertension

Nausea and Vomiting (N&V)

- Recurrent N&V in T1 occurs in 50% of pregnancies.
- If severe, can result in dehydration, electrolyte imbalance, and malnutrition.
- Management of mild cases includes:
  - Avoidance of fatty or spicy foods
  - Eating small, frequent meals
  - Inhaling peppermint oil vapors
  - Drinking ginger teas
- Management of severe cases includes:
  - Discontinuation of vitamin/mineral supplements until symptoms subside
  - Antihistamines
  - Promethazine
  - Metoclopramide
  - Intravenous droperidol

"Morning sickness" can occur day or night.

Heartburn

- Occurs in 30% of pregnancies.
- Treatment consists of:
  - Elimination of spicy/acidic foods
  - Small, frequent meals
  - Decreasing amount of liquid consumed with each meal
  - Limiting food and liquid intake a few hours prior to bedtime
  - Sleeping with head elevated on pillows
  - Utilizing liquid forms of antacids and H_2-receptor inhibitors
- Etiology is multifactorial:
  - Normal relaxation of lower esophageal sphincter
  - Mechanical forces

Constipation

- Common in pregnancy.
- Management includes:
  - Increasing intake of high-fiber foods
  - Increasing liquids
  - Use of psyllium-containing products (e.g., Metamucil)
  - Avoiding enemas, strong cathartics, and laxatives

Varicosities

- Common in pregnancy, particularly in lower extremities and vulva.
- Can lead to chronic pain and superficial thrombophlebitis.
- Management includes:
  - Avoidance of garments that constrict at the knee and upper leg
  - Use of support stockings
  - Increased periods of rest with elevation of the lower extremities

If thrombosis of a hemorrhoid occurs, clot excision should be attempted to alleviate pain and swelling.

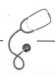

Most hemorrhoids improve after delivery.

Hemorrhoidectomy can be performed safely during pregnancy if necessary.

Rhythmic cramping pains originating in the back may signify preterm labor.

Hypercoagulable state and mechanical compression of venous blood flow to extremities leads to increased risk of thrombosis.

Hemorrhoids

- Varicosities of the rectal veins are common in pregnancy.
- Management includes:
  - Cool sitz baths
  - Stool softeners
  - Increased fluid and fiber intake to prevent constipation
  - Hemorrhoidal ointment to decrease swelling, itching, and discomfort
  - Topical anesthetic spray for the severe pain of thrombosed hemorrhoids

Leg Cramps

- Occur in 50% of pregnant women, typically at night and in T3.
- Most commonly occur in the calves.
- Massage and stretching of the affected muscle groups is recommended.

Backache

- Typically progressive in pregnancy (30–50%).
- Management includes:
  - Minimizing time standing
  - Wearing a support belt over the lower abdomen
  - Acetaminophen for pain as needed
  - Exercises to increase back strength
  - Supportive shoes and avoidance of high heels
  - Gentle back massage

Round Ligament Pain

- Sharp, bilateral or unilateral groin pain.
- Frequently occurs in T2.
- May increase with sudden movement/change in position.
- May be alleviated by patient getting on hands and knees with head on floor and buttocks in air.

Sexual Relations

- There are no restrictions during the normal pregnancy.
- Nipple stimulation, vaginal penetration, and orgasm may cause release of oxytocin and prostaglandins, resulting in uterine contractions.
- Contraindications:
  - Ruptured membranes
  - Placenta previa
  - Preterm labor

Employment

- Work activities that increase risk of falls/trauma should be avoided.
- Exposure to toxins/chemicals should be avoided.

Travel

- If prolonged sitting is involved, the patient should attempt to stretch her lower extremities and walk for 10 minutes every 2 hours.
- The patient should bring a copy of her medical record.
- Wear seat belt when riding in car.
- Airplane travel in pressurized cabin presents no additional risk to the pregnant woman (if uncomplicated pregnancy). Air travel is not recommended after 35 weeks.
- In underdeveloped areas or when traveling abroad, the usual precautions regarding ingestion of unpurified water and raw foods should be taken.

Immunizations

General principles:

- Delay vaccines until after T1 to avoid potential teratogenicity.
- Risk from vaccines is generally small. Always consider whether risk of the disease is worse than the risk of the vaccine.
- Viral vaccines may be safely given to the children of pregnant women.
- Immune globulins are safe in pregnancy and are recommended for women exposed to measles, hepatitis A and B, tetanus, varicella (chickenpox), and rabies.

Women should ideally avoid getting pregnant for 4 weeks after receiving live vaccines.

TABLE 5-2. Vaccine Safety in Pregnancy

SAFE	NOT WELL STUDIED IN PREGNANT WOMEN, SO DEFER UNTIL FURTHER RECOMMENDATIONS ISSUED	ADMINISTER ONLY IF RISK OUTWEIGHS BENEFIT	UNSAFE (LIVE)
Inactivated polio (IPV)	Human papilloma-virus (HPV)	Yellow fever	Oral polio
Inactivated typhoid	Meningococcus (MPV4)	Anthrax	Oral typhoid
Inactivated influenza	Pneumococcus (PPV)	Pertussis	Intranasal influenza
Diphtheria	Hepatitis A		Measles, mumps, rubella (MMR)
Tetanus			Varicella
Rabies			BCG
Meningococcus (MPSV4)			Shingles
Hepatitis B			

WHEN TO CALL THE PHYSICIAN

- Vaginal bleeding
- Leakage of fluid from the vagina
- Rhythmic abdominal cramping of > 6/hr that does not improve with hydration and lying supine
- Progressive and prolonged abdominal pain
- Fever and chills
- Dysuria
- Prolonged vomiting with inability to hold down liquids or solids for > 24 hours
- Progressive, severe headache; visual changes; or generalized edema
- Pronounced decrease in frequency or intensity of fetal movements

Intrapartum

Three Stages of Labor	58
True Labor versus False Labor	59
Blood Facts about the Uterus	59
Clinical Signs of Labor	60
Assessment of the Laboring Patient	60
Cervical Exam	62
Assessment of the Fetus	63
Cardinal Movements of Labor	68
Standard Method of Delivery	70
Management of Low-Risk Patients	72
Management of High-Risk Pregnancies	73
Fetal Heart Rate Patterns	75
Abnormal Labor Patterns	79
Induction of Labor	79
Cesarean Delivery	80
Vaginal Birth after Cesarean Delivery (VBAC)	81
Pain Control during Labor and Delivery	82
Pelvic Types	86

Intrapartum

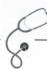

Duration of labor is typically shorter in the multiparous woman than in nulliparous women.

There are **three stages of labor,** and **two phases of stage 1.**

Remember the three "Ps" that affect the duration of the active phase:
- **Power** (strength and frequency of contractions)
- **Passenger** (size of the baby)
- **Pelvis** (size and shape of mother's pelvis)

If progress during the active phase is slower than these figures, evaluation for adequacy of uterine contractions, fetal malposition, or cephalopelvic disproportion should be done.

The successive stages of labor are illustrated in Figure 6-1.

First Stage

The first stage of labor begins with onset of **labor** (uterine contractions of sufficient frequency, intensity, and duration to result in effacement and dilation of the cervix), and ends when the cervix is fully/completely dilated to 10 cm.

The first stage of labor consists of two phases:

1. **Latent phase:** Begins with the onset of labor and ends at approximately 4 cm cervical dilation.

    Average Duration (Variable)
    - Nulliparous: 20 hours
    - Multiparous: 14 hours

2. **Active phase:** Rapid dilation. Begins at 4 cm dilation and ends at 10 cm.

Active phase is further classified according to the rate of cervical dilation: **Acceleration phase, phase of maximum slope,** and **deceleration phase.**

Fetal descent begins at 7 to 8 cm of dilation in nulliparas and becomes most rapid after 8 cm.

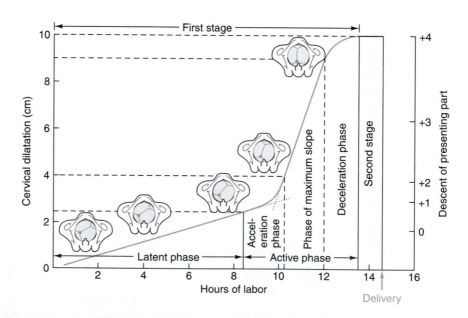

FIGURE 6-1. Schematic illustration of progress of rotation of occipitoanterior presentation in the successive stages of labor.

(Reproduced, with permission, from DeCherney AH, Pernoll ML. *Current Obstetric & Gynecologic Diagnosis & Treatment.* Norwalk, CT: Appleton & Lange, 1994: 211.)

Average duration of cervical dilation from 4 to 10 cm (minimal normal rate):
- Nulliparous: 1.2 cm/hr
- Multiparous: 1.5 cm/hr

Second Stage

The second stage of labor is the stage of **fetal expulsion.** It begins when the cervix is fully dilated and ends with the delivery of the fetus.

Average Pattern of Fetal Descent
- Nulliparous: 2 hours (3 if epidural)
- Multiparous: 1 hour (2 if epidural)

Third Stage

The main event of the third stage is placental separation. It begins immediately after the delivery of the fetus and ends with the delivery of the fetal and placental membranes.

Duration

Usually < 10 minutes; considered prolonged if > 30 minutes.

The three signs of placental separation are:

1. Gush of blood from vagina
2. Umbilical cord lengthening
3. Fundus of the uterus rises up and becomes firm

Abnormalities of the second stage may be either protraction or arrest of descent (the fetal head descends < 1 cm/hr in a nullipara and < 2 cm/hr in a multipara).

If 30 minutes have passed without placental extrusion, manual removal of the placenta may be required.

TRUE LABOR VERSUS FALSE LABOR

False Labor (Braxton Hicks Contractions)
Occur at irregular intervals
Intensity remains the same
Discomfort in lower abdomen
No cervical changes
Relieved by medications

True Labor
Occur at regular intervals that shorten
Increase in intensity
Discomfort in back and lower abdomen
Cervix changes
NOT relieved by medications

What are the three signs of placental separation?
1. Gush of blood
2. Umbilical cord lengthening
3. Fundus of uterus rises and firms

BLOOD FACTS ABOUT THE UTERUS

- Blood supply to the uterus: Uterine and ovarian arteries.
- Normal blood flow to nonpregnant uterus: 100 cc/min.
- Normal blood flow to 17-week uterus: 500 cc/min (intrauterine growth retardation occurs if flow is less).
- Normal blood loss for normal vaginal delivery: 300–500 mL.
- Normal blood loss for normal C-section: 800–1,000 mL.

Bloody Show

Discharge of small amount of blood-tinged mucus from vagina (mucous plug).

Spontaneous rupture of membranes (SROM) most often occurs during the course of active labor.

Rupture of Membranes (ROM)

ROM is characterized by sudden gush of nearly colorless fluid. ROM can be diagnosed with pool, nitrazine, and fern tests (described in PROM section).

ASSESSMENT OF THE LABORING PATIENT

Initial Assessment

History and Physical

Patients without prenatal care require a complete H&P, and those with prenatal care require an update and focused physical. Prenatal record should be obtained when possible.

Labs

Treatment of group B strep infection: IV penicillin during labor.

- Patients without prenatal care require:
  - Complete blood count (CBC).
  - Blood type and crossmatch.
  - Rh determination.
  - Urinalysis (to look for UTI).
  - Group B streptococcus testing.

Crucial Information for a Laboring Patient

The following information should always be obtained from a laboring patient:
- Time of onset and frequency of contractions.
- Status of fetal membranes.
- Presence/absence of vaginal bleeding.
- Notation of fetal activity.
- History of allergies.
- How long ago patient consumed food or liquids and how much.
- Use of medications.
- Risk status assignment (high or low).

What can cause a false-positive nitrazine test?
- Vaginal infections with *Trichomonas vaginalis*
- Blood
- Semen

Vaginal Exam (VE)

Perform a sterile speculum exam if:
- Rupture of membranes is suspected.
- The patient is in preterm labor.
- Signs of placenta previa are evident.

Otherwise, a digital VE may be performed.

The following must be assessed:

STATUS OF AMNIOTIC FLUID AND MEMBRANES

A sterile speculum is used to look for fluid in the posterior vaginal fornix (**pool test**), which determines if ROM has occurred.

Fluid may be collected on a swab for further study if the source of fluid is unclear:

- **Ferning test** (high estrogen content of amniotic fluid causes fern pattern on slide when allowed to air dry):
    - Crystallization/arborization is due to interaction of amniotic fluid proteins and salts.
    - Confirms ROM in 85–98% of cases.
- **Nitrazine test**: Nitrazine paper is pH sensitive and turns blue in the presence of amniotic fluid:
    - Amniotic fluid (pH = 7.15) is more alkaline than vaginal secretions.
    - 90–98% accurate.

Vernix: The fatty substance consisting of desquamated epithelial cells and sebaceous matter that normally covers the skin of the term fetus.
Meconium: A dark green fecal material that accumulates in the fetal intestines and is discharged at or near the time of birth.

Fluid should also be examined for meconium.

- The presence of meconium in the amniotic fluid may indicate fetal stress.
- Meconium staining is more common in term and postterm pregnancies than in preterm pregnancies.
- Meconium aspiration syndrome (MAS) can occur → infant tachypnea, costal retractions, cyanosis, coarse breath sounds, etc.
- Prevent MAS via amnioinfusion intrapartum and suction postpartum.

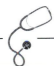

The level of the presenting part is described in relation to the ischial spines, which are designated as level 0.

STATION

Station describes the degree of descent of the fetal head (or presenting part) in relation to ischial spines.

Terminology (Two Systems)

1. The ischial spine is zero station, and the areas above and below are divided into thirds. Above the ischial spines are stations −3, −2, and −1, with −3 being the furthest above the ischial spines and −1 being closest. Positive stations describe fetal descent below the ischial spines. +3 station is at the level of the introitus, and +1 is just past the ischial spines.
2. Very similar except that the areas above and below the ischial spines are divided by centimeters, up to 5 cm above and 5 cm below. Above are five stations or centimeters: −5, −4, −3, −2, and −1, with −5 being the 5 cm above the ischial spines and −1 being 1 cm above. Positive stations describe fetal descent below the ischial spines. +5 station is at the level of the introitus, and +1 is 1 cm past the ischial spines.

If the fetus is vertex, the presenting part should be measured at the *biparietal diameter (BPD)*, not at the tip-top of the head, which may simply be caput and not the head at all. So when the *BPD* is at the level of the ischial spines, the station is 0.

THE FETAL SKULL

The top of the fetal skull is composed of five bones: two frontal, two parietal, and one occipital. The anterior fontanel lies where the two frontal and two parietal meet, and the posterior fontanel lies where the two parietal meet the occipital bone.

Anterior fontanel: bigger diamond shape
Posterior fontanel: smaller triangle shape

There are four parameters of the cervix that are examined: effacement, consistency, dilation, and position.

EFFACEMENT

Effacement describes the **length of the cervix.** With labor, the cervix thins out and softens, and the length is reduced. The normal length is 3–4 cm.

- *Terminology:* When the cervical length shrinks by 50% (to around 2 cm), it is said to be 50% effaced. When the cervix becomes as thin as the adjacent lower uterine segment, it is 100% effaced.
- *Determination of effacement:* Palpate with finger and estimate the length from the internal to external os.

DILATION

Dilation describes the size of the opening of the cervix at the external os.

- *Ranges:* Ranges from closed or zero to fully dilated (10 cm). The presenting part of a term-sized infant can usually pass through a cervix that is fully dilated.
- *Determination of dilation:* The examining finger is swept from the margin of the cervix on one side to the opposite side.

CERVICAL POSITION

Position describes the location of cervix with respect to the fetal presenting part. It is classified as one of the following:

- **Posterior:** Difficult to palpate because it is behind the fetus, and usually high in the pelvis.
- **Midposition.**
- **Anterior:** Easy to palpate, low in pelvis.

During labor, the cervical position usually progresses from posterior to anterior.

CERVICAL CONSISTENCY

Consistency ranges from firm to soft. Soft indicates onset of labor.

Bishop Score

- A scoring system that helps determine the status of the cervix—is it favorable or unfavorable for successful delivery?
- If induction of labor is indicated, the status of the cervix must be evaluated to help determine the method of labor induction that will be utilized.

See Table 6-1 and section on Labor Induction.

A score of ≥ 8 indicates that the probability of vaginal delivery after labor induction is similar to that after spontaneous labor.

HIGH-YIELD FACTS

Intrapartum

TABLE 6-1. Bishop Scoring System

Factor	0 Points	1 Point	2 Points	3 Points
Dilation (cm)	Closed	1–2	3–4	5–6
Effacement (%)	0–30	40–50	60–70	80
Station[a]	−3	−2	−1 to 0	+1 to +3
Consistency	Firm	Medium	Soft	—
Position	Posterior	Midposition	Anterior	—

[a] Station reflects −3 to +3 scale.

ASSESSMENT OF THE FETUS

Leopold Maneuvers

Leopold maneuvers are begun in midpregnancy through labor to assess the fetus and maternal abdomen (Figure 6-2). Consist of four parts:

- *First maneuver* answers the question: "What fetal part occupies the fundus?"
- *Second maneuver* answers the question: "On what side is the fetal back?"
- *Third maneuver* answers the question: "What fetal part lies over the pelvic inlet?"
- *Fourth maneuver* answers the question: "On which side is the cephalic prominence?"

Four aspects of the fetus are described from the Leopold maneuvers:
- Lie
- Presentation
- Position
- Attitude

LIE

Lie describes the relation of the long axis of the fetus to that of the mother. A **longitudinal** (99% of term or near term births) lie can be vertex (head first) or breech (buttocks first).

PRESENTATION/PRESENTING PART

Presentation describes the portion of the fetus that is foremost within the birth canal. It is normally determined by palpating through the cervix on vaginal examination.

- If the lie is longitudinal, the presentation is either the head (cephalic) or buttocks (breech). One type of cephalic presentation is the **vertex presentation** in which the posterior fontanel is the presenting part. This is considered normal.
- If the lie is transverse, the shoulder is the presenting part.

HIGH-YIELD FACTS

Intrapartum

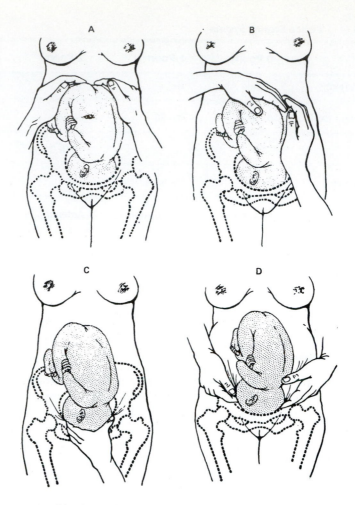

FIGURE 6-2. Leopold maneuvers.

Determining fetal presentation (A and B), position (C), and engagement (D). (Reproduced, with permission, from Pernoll ML. *Benson & Pernoll's Handbook of Obstetrics and Gynecology*, 10th ed. New York: McGraw-Hill, 2001: 159.)

Interpreting Fetal Positions: Imagine the mother lying in the anatomical position and the baby's occiput in relation to her body. You are at the end of the bed looking between mom's legs. Figure 6-3 represents the mother's birth canal with the fetal head inside in various positions as you look at the fetal head.

FETAL POSITIONS

Position refers to the relation of the presenting part to the right (R) or left (L) side of the birth canal and its direction anteriorly (A), transversely (T), or posteriorly (P).

For a cephalic occipital presentation, the position can be described in the following ways:

- Occipital anterior (OA)
- Occipital posterior (OP)
- Left occipital anterior (LOA)
- Left occipital posterior (LOP)
- Left occipital transverse (LOT)
- Right occipital anterior (ROA)
- Right occipital posterior (ROP)
- Right occipital transverse (ROT)

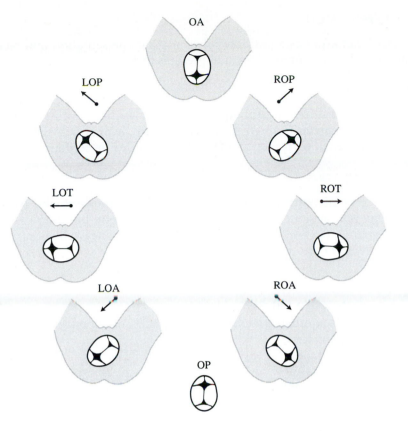

FIGURE 6-3. Vertex presentations.

FETAL ATTITUDE AND POSTURE

In the later months of pregnancy, the fetus assumes a characteristic posture ("attitude/habitus"), which typically describes the position of the arms, legs, spine, neck, and face.

Normal Presentation

VERTEX PRESENTATION (OCCIPITAL PRESENTATION)

Vertex presentation is usual (96% of at or near term presentations). The head is flexed so that the chin is in contact with the chest. The **posterior fontanel** is the presenting part.

Malpresentations

FACE PRESENTATION

In face presentation (0.3% of presentations at or near term), the fetal neck is sharply extended so the occiput is in contact with the fetal back. The face is the presenting part. Diagnosis is made by palpation of the fetal face on vaginal exam.

Vaginal delivery is possible only if the fetus is mentum anterior; mentum posterior cannot deliver vaginally → cesarean section.

SINCIPUT PRESENTATION

The fetal head assumes a position between vertex presentation and face presentation so that the anterior fontanel presents first.

BROW PRESENTATION

The fetal head assumes a position such that the eyebrows present first. This forces a large diameter through the pelvis; usually, vaginal delivery is possible only if the presentation is converted to a face or vertex presentation.

BREECH PRESENTATIONS

In breech presentations, the presenting fetal part is the buttocks. Normally, the delivery is C-section. Incidence: 3.5% at or near term but much greater in early pregnancy (14%). Those found in early pregnancy will often spontaneously convert to vertex as term approaches.

Risk Factors

- Low birth weight (20–30% of breeches)
- Congenital anomalies such as hydrocephalus or anencephaly
- Uterine anomalies
- Multiple gestation
- Placenta previa
- Hydramnios, oligohydramnios
- Multiparity

Diagnosis can be made by:
- Leopold maneuvers
- Ultrasound
- Vaginal exam

Types of Breech (see Figure 6-4)

- **Frank breech (65%):** The thighs are flexed (bent forward) and the legs are extended (straight) over the anterior surfaces of the body (feet are in front of the head or face).
- **Complete breech (25%):** The thighs are flexed (bent) on the abdomen and the legs are flexed (folded) as well.
- **Incomplete (footling) breech (10%):** One or both of the hips are not flexed so that a foot lies below.

Management

- Normally, **C-section** is the form of delivery.
- **External cephalic version:** This is maneuvering the infant to a vertex position. Can be done only if breech is diagnosed before onset of labor and the GA > 37 weeks. The success rate is 75%, and the risks are placental abruption or cord compression.

SHOULDER DYSTOCIA

Shoulder dystocia occurs when, after the fetal head has been delivered, the fetal shoulder is impacted behind the pubic symphysis.

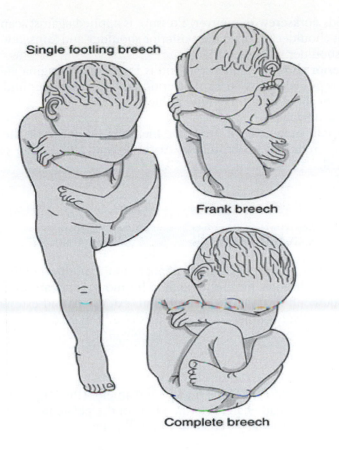

Single footling breech

Frank breech

Complete breech

FIGURE 6-4. Breech presentations.

(Reproduced, with permission, from Pernoll ML. *Benson and Pernoll's Handbook of Obstetrics & Gynecology*, 10th ed. New York: McGraw-Hill, 2001.)

Risk Factors

- Macrosomia
- Gestational diabetes
- Maternal obesity
- Post-term delivery
- Prolonged stage 2 of labor

Complications

- Fetal humeral/clavicular fracture
- Brachial plexus nerve injuries
- Hypoxia/death

Treatment

Several maneuvers can be done to displace the shoulder impaction:
- **Suprapubic pressure** on maternal abdomen.
- **McRoberts maneuver:** Maternal thighs are sharply flexed against maternal abdomen. This decreases the angle between the sacrum and spine and may dislodge fetal shoulder.

- **Woods corkscrew maneuver:** Pressure is applied against scapula of posterior shoulder to rotate the posterior shoulder and "unscrew" the anterior shoulder.
- **Posterior shoulder delivery:** Hand is inserted into vagina and posterior arm is pulled across chest, delivering posterior shoulder and displacing anterior shoulder from behind pubic symphysis.
- **Break clavicle.**
- **Zavanelli maneuver:** If the above measures do not work, the fetal head can be returned to the uterus. At this point, a C-section can be performed.

Engagement indicates that the pelvic inlet of the maternal bony pelvis is sufficiently large to allow descent of the fetal head.

Engagement is measured by palpation of the presenting part of the occiput.

Descent occurs throughout the passage through the birth canal, as does flexion of the fetal head.

CARDINAL MOVEMENTS OF LABOR

The cardinal movements of labor are changes in the position of the fetal head during passage through the birth canal. The movements are as follows: engagement, descent, flexion, internal rotation, extension, and external rotation (restitution). Delivery of the shoulders follows (see Figure 6-5).

Engagement

Engagement is the descent of the biparietal diameter (the largest transverse diameter of the fetal head, 9.5 cm) to the plane of the pelvic inlet. Often occurs before the onset of true labor, especially in nulliparas.

Descent

Descent is the fetal head passing down into the pelvis. It occurs in a discontinuous fashion. The greatest rate of descent occurs in the deceleration phase of the first stage of labor and during the second stage of labor.

Flexion

Flexion refers to the chin-to-chest position that the fetus takes. This passive motion facilitates the presentation of the smallest possible diameter of the fetal head to the birth canal.

Internal Rotation

Internal rotation refers to the fetal occiput gradually rotating toward the pubic symphysis.

Extension

Extension moves the occiput toward the fetal back:
- Occurs after the fetus has descended to the level of the maternal vulva.
- This descent brings the base of the occiput into contact with the inferior margin of the symphysis pubis, where the birth canal curves upward.

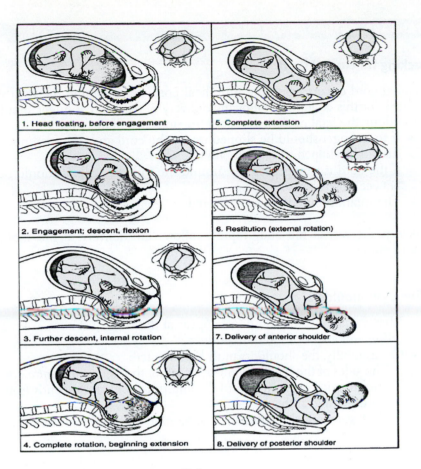

1. Head floating, before engagement

5. Complete extension

2. Engagement; descent, flexion

6. Restitution (external rotation)

3. Further descent, internal rotation

7. Delivery of anterior shoulder

4. Complete rotation, beginning extension

8. Delivery of posterior shoulder

FIGURE 6-5. Cardinal movements of labor.

(Reproduced, with permission, from Cunningham FG et al. *Williams Obstetrics*, 22nd ed. New York: McGraw-Hill, 2005: 418.)

- The fetal head is delivered by extension from the flexed to the extended position, thus curving under and past the pubic symphysis.

External Rotation (Restitution)

External rotation occurs after delivery of the head, when the fetus resumes its normal "face-forward" position with the occiput and spine lying in the same plane.

External rotation is completed by rotation of the fetal body to the transverse position (i.e., one shoulder is anterior behind the pubic symphysis and the other is posterior).

Expulsion

After external rotation, further descent brings the anterior shoulder to the level of the pubic symphysis. The shoulder is delivered under the pubic symphysis and then the rest of the body is quickly delivered.

The anterior shoulder is the one closest to the superior portions of the vagina, while the posterior shoulder is closest to the perineum and anus.

Checking for Nuchal Cord

A nuchal cord occurs when the umbilical cord wraps around the fetal neck. To check for this condition, following delivery of the head, a finger should be passed along the fetal neck to ascertain the presence of the cord.

- If so, a finger should be slipped under the cord and, if loose enough, it should be slipped over the infant's head.
- If the cord is wrapped tightly around the infant's neck, it should be cut between two clamps.
- The infant should then be delivered.

Typically, the rest of the body rapidly follows the delivery of the shoulders without effort.

Delivery of Shoulders

- Most frequently, the shoulders appear at the vulva just after external rotation and are born spontaneously.
- Occasionally, the shoulders must be extracted:
  - The sides of the head are grasped with both hands and *gentle* downward traction is applied until the anterior shoulder descends from under the pubic arch.
  - Next, *gentle* upward traction is applied to deliver the posterior shoulder.

Vaginal Lacerations

The perineum and anus become stretched and thin, which results in increased risk of spontaneous laceration and anterior tears involving the urethra and labia.

FIRST DEGREE

- Involve the fourchette, perineal skin, and vaginal mucosa, but *not* the underlying fascia and muscle.
- Repair: Absorbable sutures (e.g., 3-0 vicryl).

SECOND DEGREE

- First degree plus the fascia and muscle of the perineal body but *not* the rectal sphincter.
- Repair: Done in layers, sometimes using a crown stitch to bring the perineal body together.

THIRD DEGREE

- Second degree plus involvement of the anal sphincter.
- Repair: Repair anal sphincter with interrupted sutures and repair vagina as in second-degree laceration.

- Extend through the rectal mucosa to expose the lumen of the rectum.
- Repair: Same as third-degree repair plus careful repair of anal mucosa (e.g., with 4-0 vicryl).

Proper repair of fourth-degree laceration is important to prevent future maternal problems (e.g., fecal incontinence, rectovaginal fistula).

Episiotomy

An episiotomy is the incision of the perineum and/or labia to aid delivery. There are two types:

1. **Midline:** The incision is made in the midline from the posterior fourchette. Most common. Increases the risk of a fourth-degree lacration.
2. **Mediolateral:** The incision is oblique starting from 5 o'clock or 7 o'clock position of the vagina. Causes more infection and pain.

Indications

- Risk of perineal rupture
- Shoulder dystocia
- Breech delivery
- Forceps/vacuum delivery

Postdelivery Tasks

1. Clear the nasopharynx:
   - To minimize infant aspiration of amniotic fluid debris and blood that may occur once the thorax is delivered and the baby can inspire.
   - Use a bulb syringe to aspirate the mouth and nares.
2. Clamping and cutting the cord:
   - The umbilical cord is clamped by two instruments and cut in between.
   - The infant is handed to the pediatrician/nurse/assistant for examination.
   - A sample of cord blood is taken from the umbilical cord that remains attached to the placenta.

Squeeze the bulb-suction between fingers *first*, then place in fetal mouth/nares.

Postdelivery Uterine Exam

- The height and consistency of the uterine fundus are ascertained.
- A moderate amount of bleeding is normal.

Postdelivery, the uterus should be firm and contracted, like a ball.

Placental Separation

Signs

1. Uterus becomes globular and more firm.
2. There is often a sudden gush of blood.
3. The uterus rises in the abdomen due to the bulk of the placenta, which has (separated) passed down into the lower uterine segment and vagina.
4. The umbilical cord protrudes farther out of the vagina, indicating descent of the placenta.

Signs of placental separation typically occur within 5 minutes of infant delivery.

Delivery of the Placenta

- Pressure is applied to the body of the uterus (pushed cephalad with the abdominal hand) as the umbilical cord is held slightly taut.
- This maneuver is repeated until the placenta reaches the introitus.
- As the placenta passes to the introitus, pressure on the uterus is stopped.
- The placenta is gently lifted away from the introitus.
- The maternal surface of the placenta should be examined to ensure that no placental fragments are left in the uterus.

Postdelivery Hemostasis

After the uterus has been emptied and the placenta delivered, hemostasis must be achieved:

- The primary mechanism is myometrial contraction → vasoconstriction.
- Oxytocin (Pitocin) is administered in the third stage of labor → myometrial contractions → reduces maternal blood loss.

Dystocia

Dystocia literally means difficult labor and is characterized by abnormally slow progress of labor.

Causes

1. Abnormalities of the expulsive forces:
   - Uterine dysfunction → uterine forces insufficiently strong or inappropriately coordinated to efface and dilate cervix.
   - Inadequate voluntary muscle effort during second stage of labor.
2. Abnormalities of presentation, position, or fetal development.
3. Abnormalities of the maternal bony pelvis.
4. Abnormalities of the birth canal.

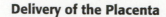

MANAGEMENT OF LOW-RISK PATIENTS

Monitoring Uterine Activity

UTERINE CONTRACTIONS

Uterine activity is monitored by internal or external uterine pressure monitors. Pressure is calculated in *Montevideo units*, calculated by increases in uterine pressure above baseline (8–12 mm Hg) multiplied by contraction frequency per 10 minutes. If you have time, don't multiply—add every contraction.

UTERINE PRESSURE INCREASES AND STAGES OF LABOR

Uterine contractions in the first stage of labor increase progressively in intensity from 25 to 50 mm Hg, and the frequency increases from three to five contractions per 10 minutes.

Contractions in the second stage increase further (aided by maternal bearing down) to 80–100 mm Hg, and the frequency increases to five to six per 10 minutes.

Vaginal Exams

Vaginal examinations should be kept to the minimum required for the evaluation of a normal labor pattern, for example, every 4 hours in latent phase and every 2 hours in active phase. Sterile gloves and lubricant should be used.

Fetal Heart Rate Monitoring

The fetal heart rate (FHR) can be measured in two ways:

1. Intermittent auscultation with a fetal stethoscope or Doppler ultrasonic device.
2. Continuous electronic monitoring of the FHR and uterine contractions.

FIRST STAGE OF LABOR

Fetal heart rate should be recorded every 30 minutes (immediately after uterine contractions).

SECOND STAGE OF LABOR

Fetal heart rate should be recorded every 15 minutes (immediately after uterine contractions).

Maternal Vital Signs

Maternal blood pressure and pulse should be evaluated and recorded every 10 minutes.

Other Considerations

Usually, oral intake is limited to small sips of water, ice chips, or hard candies.

Inhalation anesthesia may be needed for cesarean delivery or for management of complications in the third stage of labor. Thus, consumption of foods or liquids can cause aspiration.

MANAGEMENT OF HIGH-RISK PREGNANCIES

Same as above with addition of the following:

Continuous Electronic Fetal Monitoring

Continuous electronic fetal monitoring should be done with evaluation of tracing every 15 minutes during first stage and every 5 minutes during second stage. It can be done in either of the following two ways:

1. *Internal electronic FHR monitoring:* Internal FHR monitoring is done with a bipolar spiral electrode attached to fetal scalp, which detects the peak R-wave voltage of the fetal electrocardiogram.
2. *External (indirect) electronic FHR monitoring:* FHR is detected through the maternal abdominal wall with a transducer that emits ultrasound. Uterine contractions are also detected.

Nonstress Test

The nonstress test (NST) is the first assessment of fetal well-being:

- The mother is placed in a left lateral position.
- A continuous FHR tracing is obtained using external Doppler equipment.
- The heart rate changes that result from the fetal movements are determined:
    - A normal fetal response during each fetal movement is an acceleration in fetal heart rate of ≥ 15 bpm above the baseline for at least 15 seconds.
    - If at least two such accelerations occur in a 20-minute interval, the fetus is deemed healthy and the test is **reactive.**
- If an NST is **nonreactive,** it should be followed by a biophysical profile (BPP) or contraction stress test.

Contraction Stress Test

- Not routinely used due to risks.
- Evaluate FHR response to contractions.
- Need to induce contractions with oxytocin or nipple stimulation.

Biophysical Profile

The physiologic basis for using the BPP lies in the fact that coordinated fetal activities (i.e., breathing and movement) require an intact, nonhypoxic central nervous system.

A BPP uses ultrasonography and cardiotocography to ascertain fetal well-being by assessing the following five parameters:

1. Fetal breathing movements (chest wall movements)
2. Fetal activity (gross trunk or limb movements)
3. Amniotic fluid index
4. Fetal tone (flexion and extension of an extremity)
5. Reactivity (nonstress test)

A score of 0 or 2 is given for each parameter and a normal profile equals 8–10.

Amniotic Fluid Index

Amniotic fluid plays an important role in fetal lung development protection against trauma and infection. The amniotic fluid index (AFI) is examined in the BPP and reflects the volume of amniotic fluid. The calculation of AFI is as follows: The maternal abdomen is divided into quadrants, and with ultrasound, the maximum vertical pocket of each quadrant is measured in centimeters and added.

Normal Amniotic Fluid Index

- Maximum amniotic fluid is at 28 weeks—800 mL.
- After 28 weeks, amniotic fluid decreases.
- At 40 weeks, amniotic fluid is at 500 mL.

Abnormal Amniotic Fluid Index

- **Oligohydramnios** is < 5 amniotic fluid index.
  - Most common cause: Rupture of membranes.
  - Associated with intrauterine growth retardation (IUGR) in 60% of cases. Consider genitourinary malformations, infections.
- **Polyhydramnios** is > 20 amniotic fluid index, or 2 L.

FETAL HEART RATE PATTERNS

Important Definitions

- **Hypoxemia:** Decreased oxygen content in blood.
- **Hypoxia:** Decreased level of oxygen in tissue.
- **Acidemia:** Increased concentration of hydrogen ions in the blood.
- **Acidosis:** Increased concentration of hydrogen ions in tissue.
- **Asphyxia:** Hypoxia with metabolic acidosis.

Reactivity and the Normal FHR

The normal fetal heart rate is 110–160 bpm. This baseline (a "baseline" rate refers to a heart rate lasting ≥ 10 minutes) normally has frequent periodic variations above and below termed **accelerations** (increases in HR) and **decelerations** (decreases in HR) (See Table 6-2 and Figure 6-6.)

A normally reactive fetal tracing has two accelerations of at least 15 bpm greater than the baseline, lasting for at least 15 seconds, in 20 minutes. It represents intact neurohumoral cardiovascular control mechanisms and indicates that the fetus is unstressed.

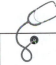

Reactive: 15-bpm increase of 15-second duration 2×/20 minutes.

TABLE 6-2. FHR Patterns

	EARLY DECELERATION	**LATE DECELERATION**	**VARIABLE DECELERATION**
Significance	Benign	Abnormal	Mild
Shape	U shaped	U shaped	Variable (often V or W shaped)
Onset	Gradual	Gradual	Abrupt
Depth	Shallow	Shallow	Variable
When	End with the uterine contraction	Start after the uterine contraction	Variable
Why	Head compression	Uteroplacental insufficiency	Cord compression and occasionally head compression
Initial treatment	None required	O$_2$, lateral decubitus position, Pitocin off, close monitoring	Amnioinfusion

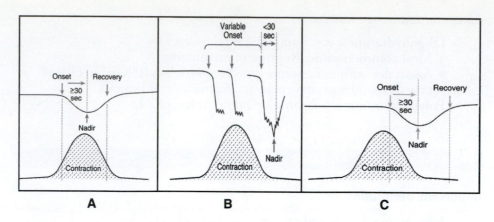

FIGURE 6-6. Features of early (A), variable (B), and late (C) decelerations on fetal heart monitoring.

(Reproduced, with permission, from Cunningham FG et al. *Williams Obstetrics*, 22nd ed. New York: McGraw-Hill, 2005: 452, 453, 454.)

A fetus < 28 weeks' GA is neurologically immature and thus is not expected to have a "reactive" FHR.

Periodic FHR Changes

Periodic FHR changes refers to accelerations and decelerations related to uterine contractions (i.e., contraction stress test).

DECELERATIONS

Decelerations during labor have different meaning depending on when they occur in relation to contractions.

Early Decelerations

Early decelerations are *normal* and due to head compression during contractions. The timing of onset, peak, and end coincides with the timing of the contraction. The degree of deceleration is proportional to the contraction strength. The effect is regulated by vagal nerve activation. No intervention is necessary.

Late Decelerations

Late decelerations are *abnormal* and are due to **uteroplacental insufficiency** (not enough blood) during contractions. They begin at the peak of contraction and end slowly after the contraction has stopped. Can follow epidural (hypotension) or uterine hyperstimulation.

The lateral recumbent position (either side) is best for maximizing cardiac output and uterine blood flow. (In the supine position, the vena cava and aortoiliac vessels may be compressed by the gravid uterus.)

Intervention
- **Change maternal position to the lateral recumbent position.**
- **Give oxygen by face mask.**
- **Stop oxytocin (Pitocin) infusion.**
- Provide an IV fluid bolus.
- Consider tocolysis.
- Monitor maternal blood pressure.
- If persist > 30 minutes or worsen, fetal scalp blood pH should be obtained and C-section considered.

Variable Decelerations

Variable decelerations are *abnormal* and can be mild or severe. They are due to **cord compression** and sometimes **head compression**. They can occur at any time. If they are repetitive, suspicion is high for the cord to be wrapped around the neck or under the arm of the fetus.

Intervention
- **Amnioinfusion:** Infuse normal saline into the uterus through the intrauterine pressure catheter to alleviate cord compression.
- Change maternal position to side/Trendelenburg position.
- Deliver fetus with forceps or C-section if worsening.

FETAL TACHYCARDIA

Mild = 161 to 180 bpm
Severe = ≥ 181

Fetal tachycardia may indicate intrauterine infection, severe fetal hypoxia, congenital heart disease, or maternal fever.

BEAT-TO-BEAT VARIABILITY (BTBV)

- **The single most important characteristic of the baseline FHR.**
- Variation of successive beats in the FHR BTBV is controlled primarily by the autonomic nervous system, thus an important index of fetal central nervous system (CNS) integrity.
- At < 28 weeks' GA, the fetus is neurologically immature; thus, decreased variability is expected.

Short-Term Variability (STV)
- Reflects instantaneous beat-to-beat (R wave to R wave) changes in FHR.
- The *roughness* (STV present) or *smoothness* (STV absent) of the FHR tracing.
- May be decreased/absent due to alterations in the CNS or inadequate fetal oxygenation.

Long-Term Variability (LTV)
- Describes the oscillatory changes that occur in 1 minute.
- Results in waviness of baseline.
- Normal = 3–6 cycles/min.

Decreases in BTBV

Beat-to-beat variability decreases with:
- Fetal acidemia
- Fetal asphyxia
- Maternal acidemia
- Drugs (narcotics, $MgSO_4$, barbiturates, etc.)

Increases in BTBV

Beat-to-beat variability increases with mild fetal hypoxemia.

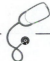

Variable decelerations are abnormal.
They are classified as:
Mild
- Lasts < 30 sec and depth > 70 to 80 bpm

Moderate
- Lasts 30 to 60 sec and depth < 70 to 80 bpm
OR
- Lasts > 60 sec and depth = 70 to 80 bpm

Severe
- Lasts > 60 sec and depth < 70 bpm

May signify fetal **acidemia.**

If an FHR of 160 bpm lasts for ≥ 10 minutes, then tachycardia is present.

No BTBV = **fetal acidosis,** and the fetus must be delivered immediately.

BTBV can be reliably determined only with internal FHR monitoring (fetal scalp electrode).

Short-term variability is thought to be the most important predictor of fetal outcome.

Prolonged Decelerations

Isolated decelerations that last 2–10 minutes. Causes include:
- Cervical examinations
- Uterine hyperactivity
- Maternal hypotension leading to transient fetal hypoxia
- Umbilical cord compression

Management

- Stop oxytocin and prostaglandins.
- Change maternal position.
- Administer IV fluids.
- If mother is hypotensive, administer ephedrine/terbutaline.
- Administer maternal O_2.
- Rule out cord prolapse.

TABLE 6-3. **Abnormal Labor Patterns**

LABOR PATTERN	DIAGNOSTIC CRITERION: NULLIPARAS	DIAGNOSTIC CRITERION: MULTIPARAS	PREFERRED TREATMENT	EXCEPTIONAL TREATMENT
Prolongation disorder (prolonged latent phase)	> 20 hrs	> 14 hrs	Therapeutic rest (may be unrecognized false labor)	Oxytocin stimulation or cesarean delivery for urgent problems
Protraction disorder				
1. Protracted active phase dilatation	< 1.2 cm/hr	< 1.5 cm/hr		
2. Protracted descent	< 1 cm/hr	< 2 cm/hr	Expectant and support	Cesarean delivery for cephalopelvic disproportion (CPD)
Arrest disorders				
1. Prolonged deceleration phase	> 3 hrs	> 1 hr	Without CPD: Oxytocin	Rest if exhausted
2. Secondary arrest of dilatation	> 2 hrs	> 2 hrs		
3. Arrest of descent	> 1 hr	> 1 hr	With CPD: Cesarean delivery	Cesarean delivery
4. Failure of descent (no descent in deceleration phase or second stage of labor)	> 1 hr	> 1 hr		

- *Prolonged latent phase* (see Table 6-3).
- *Active phase abnormalities*—may be due to cephalopelvic disproportion (CPD), excessive sedation, conduction analgesia, and fetal malposition (i.e., persistent OP).
  - *Protraction disorders*—a slow rate of cervical dilation or descent
  - *Arrest disorders*—complete cessation of dilation or descent (see Table 6-3)

INDUCTION OF LABOR

Indications

When risks of pregnancy (mother or fetus) outweigh the risks of delivery. Need to confirm fetal lung maturity for "elective" inductions. No absolute indication:

- Suspicion of fetal compromise.
- Shortening of second stage (i.e., maternal benefit), heart disease, pulmonary edema, exhaustion, aneurysm.

If a deceleration has occurred without recovery after 2 minutes, an emergency C-section is required.

Maternal
- Premature ROM
- Diabetes mellitus
- Heart disease
- Prolonged labor
- Prolonged pregnancy
- Worsening/severe preeclampsia
- Post term

Fetal
- IUGR
- Abnormal fetal testing
- Infection
- Rh incompatibility
- Oligohydramnios

Relative
- Distance from hospital
- History of precipitous labor
- Weather (e.g., winter storm)

Contraindications

Maternal
- Contracted pelvis
- Prior uterine surgery (controversial)
- Classic cesarean section
- Myomectomy with endometrial cavity violation

Fetal
- Lung immaturity
- Acute distress
- Abnormal presentation

Scalp stimulation is done *between* decelerations to elicit a reactive acceleration and rule out metabolic acidosis.

Confirmation of Term

1. Documented FHT:
   - 20 weeks by nonelectronic fetoscope
   - 30 weeks by Doppler
2. 36 weeks since a positive pregnancy test at a reliable laboratory
3. Ultrasound-confirmed GA of at least 39 weeks by:
   - Crown–rump length at 6–12 weeks
   - Dating US at 13–20 weeks

HIGH-YIELD FACTS

Intrapartum

Induction Methods

OXYTOCIN

A synthetic polypeptide hormone that stimulates uterine contraction:
- Acts promptly when given intravenously. Half-life 3–5 minutes.
- Should not be employed for more than a few hours.

Complications

- Potent antidiuretic effects of oxytocin (oxytocin is related structurally and functionally to vasopressin or antidiuretic hormone) can cause water intoxication (i.e., hyponatremia), which can lead to convulsions, coma, and death.
- Risk of uterine tetanic contractions (overstimulation).

PROSTAGLANDINS

- Misoprostol, a synthetic PGE_1 analog:
  - Can be administered intravaginally or orally
  - Used for cervical ripening and induction
- PGE_2 gel and vaginal insert:
  - Both contain dinoprostone
  - Used for cervical ripening in women at or near term

MECHANICAL

- Foley
- Laminaria

CESAREAN DELIVERY

The birth of a fetus through incisions in the abdominal wall (laparotomy) and the uterine wall (hysterotomy).

Basic Types

1. Low cervical (also called low-transverse cesarean section [LTCS]):
   - Incision made in lower uterine segment
   - Most common type performed
2. Classical:
   - Vertical incision made in uterine corpus
   - Done when:
     - Lower uterine segment not developed (i.e., prematurity)
     - Fetus is transverse lie with back down

Indications

- Prior cesarean (elective; patient does not desire a trial of labor)
- Dystocia or failure to progress in labor
- Breech presentation
- Transverse lie
- Concern for fetal well-being (i.e., fetal distress)
- Uterine malformations/scars

- VBAC is associated with a small but significant risk of uterine rupture with poor outcome for mother and infant:
  - Classical uterine incision: 4–9% risk
  - Low-transverse incision: 0.2–1.5% risk
- Maternal and infant complications are also associated with an unsuccessful trial of labor.

Candidates for VBAC

- **One or two prior LTCSs.**
- Clinically adequate pelvis.
- No other uterine scars or previous rupture.
- Physician immediately available throughout active labor capable of monitoring labor and performing an emergency C-section.
- Availability of anesthesia and personnel for emergency C-section.

Contraindications to VBAC

- **Prior classical or T-shaped incision or other transfundal uterine surgery.**
- Contracted pelvis.
- Medical/obstetric complication that precludes vaginal delivery.
- Inability to perform emergency C-section because of unavailable surgeon, anesthesia, sufficient staff, or facility.

Forceps Delivery

Forceps can be used to shorten the second stage of labor when in the best interest of the fetus or the mother. The cervix must be fully dilated.

Indications

- Lack of progress for ≥ 3 hours in nullipara with regional anesthesia.
- Lack of progress for ≥ 2 hours in nullipara without regional anesthesia.
- Lack of progress for ≥ 2 hours in multipara with regional anesthesia.
- Lack of progress for ≥ 1 hours in multipara without regional anesthesia.
- Fetal distress.
- Maternal factors: Exhaustion, heart disease, pulmonary edema, aneurysm, etc.

Contraindications

- Fetal head is not engaged or is in a presentation other than vertex.
- Position of head is not precisely known.
- Membranes are not ruptured.
- Cervix is not fully dilated.
- Presence of cephalopelvic disproportion.

The skin incision that you see on the maternal abdomen does not tell you the type of uterine incision that the patient received. For example, a woman may have a classical uterine incision, but a low transverse skin incision (Pfanenstiel incision).

HIGH-YIELD FACTS

Intrapartum

Vacuum Delivery

A safe, effective alternative to forceps delivery. A term, vertex fetus is required. Delivery should not be one that will require rotation or excessive traction. Prior scalp sampling is a contraindication.

Advantages

- Simpler to apply with fewer mistakes in application.
- Less force applied to fetal head.
- Less anesthesia is necessary (local anesthetic may suffice).
- No increase in diameter of presenting head.
- Less maternal soft-tissue injury.
- Less parental concern.

Disadvantages

- Traction is applied only during contractions.
- Proper traction is necessary to avoid losing vacuum.
- Possible longer delivery than with forceps.
- Small increase in incidence of cephalohematomas.

Technique

- Ascertain that the cervix is fully dilated and the head is in low or outlet position.
- The head is then wiped clean, the labia are spread, and the cup is compressed and inserted. Pressure is applied inward and downward until contact is made with the fetal scalp. The cup should be placed over the posterior fontanel.
- A finger is swept around the cup to make sure no maternal tissue is within the cup. Suction pressure is raised to 100 mm Hg, and the location of the cup is rechecked.
- With the onset of a contraction, suction pressure is raised to a range of 380–580 mm Hg. (Negative pressure should not exceed 600 mm Hg.) Traction is applied perpendicularly to the cup, in line with the maternal axis.
- Should the cup be dislodged, the fetal scalp is to be checked before the cup is reapplied.
- When the contraction subsides, the suction pressure is reduced to 100 mm Hg.
- As the head crowns, an episiotomy may be cut but likely increases the risk of third- and fourth-degree tears. Traction is then changed to a 45-degree angle upward as the vertex clears the symphysis.
- Suction is released and the cup removed after delivery of the fetal head.
- The procedure should be discontinued if one fails to achieve extraction after 10 minutes at maximal pressure, extraction is not achieved within 30 minutes of initiation, the cup disengages three times, fetal scalp trauma is sustained, or no progress is made after three pulls.

PAIN CONTROL DURING LABOR AND DELIVERY

Three essentials of obstetrical pain relief are simplicity, safety, and preservation of fetal homeostasis.

Lower Genital Tract Innervation

During the second stage of labor, much of the pain arises from the lower genital tract:

- Painful stimuli from the lower genital tract are primarily transmitted by the pudendal nerve which passes beneath the posterior surface of the sacrospinous ligament (just as the ligament attaches to the ischial spine).
- The sensory nerve fibers of the pudendal nerve are derived from the ventral branches of the second, third, and fourth sacral nerves.

The peripheral branches of the pudendal nerve provide sensory innervation to the perineum, anus, and the medial and inferior parts of the vulva and clitoris.

Nonpharmacological Methods of Pain Control

Women who are free from fear and who have confidence in their obstetrical staff require smaller amounts of pain medication:

- An understanding of pregnancy and the birth process.
- Appropriate antepartum training in breathing.
- Appropriate psychological support (e.g., by a friend or family member).
- Considerate obstetricians and labor assistants who instill confidence.

Analgesia and Sedation

Pain relief with an opiate or opioid plus an antiemetic is typically sufficient, with **no significant risk** to the mother or infant:

- Discomfort is still felt at the acme of an effective uterine contraction but is more tolerable.
- Slight increase in uterine activity.
- Does *not* prolong labor.

Uterine contractions and cervical dilation cause discomfort.

General Anesthesia

General anesthesia should not be induced until all steps preparatory to actual delivery have been completed, so as to minimize transfer of the agent to the fetus, thereby avoiding newborn respiratory depression.

Concerns

- All anesthetic agents that depress the maternal CNS cross the placenta and depress the fetal CNS.
- General anesthetics can cause aspiration of gastric contents and particulate matter, leading to airway obstruction, pneumonitis, pulmonary edema, and/or death.

If delivery occurs within 1 hour of analgesia, neonatal depression may occur.

Regional Analgesia

Nerve blocks that provide pain relief for women in labor and delivery without loss of consciousness. Preferred agents include bupivicaine.

PUDENDAL BLOCK

- Local infiltration of the pudendal nerve with a local anesthetic agent (e.g., lidocaine).

- Allows pinching of the lower vagina and posterior vulva bilaterally without pain.
- Effective, safe, and reliable method of providing analgesia for spontaneous delivery.
- Can be used along with epidural analgesia.

Complications

Inadvertent intravascular injection will cause systemic toxicity, hematoma, infection.

PARACERVICAL BLOCK

- Agent is injected at the 3 o'clock and 9 o'clock positions around the cervix.
- Provides good relief of pain of uterine contractions during first stage of labor.
- Requires additional analgesia for delivery because the pudendal nerves are not blocked.

Complications

Fetal bradycardia (usually transient).

SPINAL (SUBARACHNOID) BLOCK

- Introduction of local anesthetic into the subarachnoid space.
- Used for uncomplicated cesarean delivery and vaginal delivery of normal women of low parity.

LOW SPINAL BLOCK

- Level of analgesia extends to the tenth thoracic dermatome (corresponds to the level of the umbilicus).
- Popular for forceps or vacuum delivery.
- Provides excellent relief of pain from uterine contractions.
- Preceded by infusion of 1 L of crystalloid solution to prevent hypotension.

HIGH SPINAL BLOCK

- A higher level of spinal blockade is necessary to at least the level of the eighth thoracic dermatome (just below the xiphoid process of the sternum).
- A larger dose of anesthetic agent is required to anesthetize the larger area, which results in increased frequency and intensity of toxic reactions.

Complications

- Maternal hypotension (common)
- Total spinal blockade
- Spinal (postpuncture) headache
- Seizures
- Bladder dysfunction

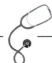

Prophylactic measures against aspiration include fasting for at least 6 hours prior to anesthesia and antacid administration before induction.

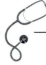

Always pull back on the syringe prior to injection of anesthetic to look for blood flow into the syringe; if positive, you are in a vessel and must reposition your needle.

Contraindications

- Severe preeclampsia
- Coagulation/hemostasis disorders
- Neurologic disorders

EPIDURAL ANALGESIA

Injection of local anesthetic into the epidural or peridural space:

- *Lumbar epidural analgesia*: Injection into a lumbar intervertebral space.
- *Caudal epidural analgesia*: Injection through the sacral hiatus and sacral canal.

Relieves pain of uterine contractions, abdominal delivery (block begins at the eighth thoracic level and extends to first sacral dermatome) or vaginal delivery (block begins from the tenth thoracic to the fifth sacral dermatome).

The spread of the anesthetic agent depends on:

1. Location of the catheter tip
2. Dose, concentration, and volume of anesthetic agent used
3. Maternal position (e.g., head up, head down, horizontal)
4. Individual anatomy of epidural space (i.e., presence of synechiae may preclude a satisfactory block)

Complications

- Inadvertent spinal blockade (puncture of dura with subarachnoid injection)
- Ineffective analgesia
- Hypotension
- Seizures

Effects on Labor

- Increased duration of labor
- Increased incidence of:
  - Chorioamnionitis
  - Low-forceps procedures
  - Cesarean deliveries
  - Maternal pyrexia

Contraindications

- Actual/anticipated serious maternal hemorrhage
- Infection at or near sites for puncture
- Suspicion of neurological disease

LOCAL INFILTRATION

Employed for delivery:

- Before episiotomy and delivery
- After delivery in the site of lacerations to be repaired
- Around the episiotomy wound if there is inadequate analgesia

When vaginal delivery is anticipated in 10 to 15 minutes, a rapidly acting agent is given through the epidural catheter to effect perineal analgesia.

HIGH-YIELD FACTS

Intrapartum

	GYNECOID	**ANDROID**	**ANTHROPOID**	**PLATYPELLOID**
	(circle)	(heart shape)	(vertical oval)	(horizontal oval)
Frequency	In 50% of all females	One third of white women; one sixth of nonwhite women	One fourth of white women; one half of nonwhite women	Rarest, < 3% of women
Inlet shape	Round	Heart shaped	Vertically oriented oval	Horizontally oriented oval
Sidewalls	Straight	Convergent	Convergent	Divergent, then convergent
Ischial spines	Not prominent (diameter ≥ 10 cm)	Prominent (diameter < 10 cm)	Prominent (diameter < 10 cm)	Not prominent (diameter > 10 cm)
Sacrum	Inclined neither anteriorly nor posteriorly	Forward and straight with little curvature	Straight = pelvis deeper than other three types	Well curved and rotated backward; short = shallow pelvis
Significance	Good prognosis for vaginal delivery	Limited posterior space for fetal head → poor prognosis for vaginal delivery	Good prognosis for vaginal delivery	Poor prognosis for vaginal delivery

HIGH-YIELD FACTS IN

Postpartum

The Puerperium of the Normal Labor and Delivery   88

Routine Postpartum Care   90

Postpartum Patient Education   92

Maternal Follow-up Care   94

Postpartum Psychiatric Disorders   95

The puerperium is the period of confinement during birth and 6 weeks after. During this time, the reproductive tract returns anatomically to a normal non-pregnant state.

Uterine Changes

INVOLUTION OF THE UTERINE CORPUS

Immediately after delivery, the fundus of the contracted uterus is slightly below the umbilicus. After the first 2 days postpartum, the uterus begins to shrink in size. Within 2 weeks, the uterus has descended into the cavity of the true pelvis.

ENDOMETRIAL CHANGES: SLOUGHING AND REGENERATION

Within 2–3 days postpartum, the remaining decidua become differentiated into two layers:

1. Superficial layer becomes necrotic, sloughs off as vaginal discharge = *lochia*.
2. Basal layer (adjacent to the myometrium) becomes new endometrium.

Placental Site Involution

Within hours after delivery, the placental site consists of many thrombosed vessels. Immediately postpartum, the placental site is the size of the palm of the hand. The site rapidly decreases in size and by 2 weeks postpartum = 3–4 cm in diameter.

Changes in Uterine Vessels

Blood vessels are obliterated by hyaline changes and replaced by new, smaller vessels.

Changes in the Cervix and Lower Uterine Segment

The external os of the cervix contracts slowly and has narrowed by the end of the first week.

The thinned-out lower uterine segment (that contained most of the fetal head) contracts and retracts over a few weeks → uterine isthmus.

Changes in the Vagina and Vaginal Outlet

Gradually diminishes in size, but rarely returns to nulliparous dimensions:
- Rugae reappear by the third week.
- The rugae become obliterated after repeated childbirth and menopause.

"Afterpains" due to uterine contraction are common and may require analgesia. They typically decrease in intensity by the third postpartum day.

Lochia is decidual tissue that contains erythrocytes, epithelial cells, and bacteria.
See Table 7-1.

TABLE 7-1. Lochia

TYPE	DESCRIPTION	WHEN OBSERVED
Lochia rubra	Red due to blood in the lochia	Days 1–3
Lochia serosa	More pale in color	Days 4–10
Lochia alba	White to yellow-white due to leukocytes and reduced fluid content	Day 11 →

Peritoneum and Abdominal Wall

The broad ligaments and round ligaments slowly relax to the nonpregnant state.

The abdominal wall is soft and flabby due to the prolonged distention and rupture of the skin's elastic fibers; resumes prepregnancy appearance in several weeks, except for silver striae.

Urinary Tract Changes

The puerperal bladder:
- Has an increased capacity
- Is relatively insensitive to intravesical fluid pressure

Hence, overdistention, incomplete bladder emptying, and excessive residual urine are common and can result in a urinary tract infection (UTI).

Between days 2 and 5 postpartum, "puerperal diuresis" typically occurs to reverse the increase in extracellular water associated with normal pregnancy.

Dilated ureters and renal pelves return to their prepregnant state from 2 to 8 weeks postpartum.

Changes in the Breasts

DEVELOPMENT OF MILK-SECRETING MACHINERY

Progesterone, estrogen, placental lactogen, prolactin, cortisol, and insulin act together to stimulate the growth and development of the milk-secreting machinery of the mammary gland:
- Midpregnancy—lobules of alveoli form lobes separated by stromal tissue, with secretion in some alveolar cells.
- T3—alveolar lobules are almost fully developed, with cells full of proteinaceous secretory material.
- Postpartum—rapid increase in cell size and in the number of secretory organelles. Alveoli distend with milk.

DEVELOPMENT OF THE MILK

At delivery, the abrupt, large decrease in progesterone and estrogen levels leads to increased production of alpha-lactalbumin, which stimulates lactose synthase, resulting in milk production.

When involution of the uterus is defective, late puerperal hemorrhage may occur.

At the completion of involution, the cervix does *not* resume its pregravid appearance:
Before childbirth, the os is a small, regular, oval opening.
After childbirth, the orifice is a transverse slit.

The uterine isthmus is located between the uterine corpus above and the internal cervical os below.

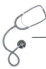

All postpartum women who cannot void should be promptly catheterized.

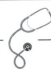

What causes fluid retention postpartum?
- *High estrogen levels* in pregnancy
- *Increased venous pressure* in the lower half of the body during pregnancy

Colostrum is a deep yellow-colored liquid secreted by the breasts that contains minerals, protein, fat, antibodies, complement, macrophages, lymphocytes, lysozymes, lactoferrin, and lactoperoxidase.

Women with extensive pituitary necrosis (Sheehan syndrome) cannot breast-feed due to the absence of prolactin.

Breast engorgement seldom persists for > 24 hours. Other causes of fever (e.g., mastitis, endometritis, UTI, thrombophlebitis) must be excluded.

Milk letdown may be provoked by the cry of the infant or inhibited by stress or fright.

COLOSTRUM

Colostrum can be expressed from the nipple by the second postpartum day and is secreted by the breasts for 5 days postpartum.

MATURE MILK AND LACTATION

Colostrum is then gradually converted to mature milk by 4 weeks postpartum. Subsequent lactation is primarily controlled by the repetitive stimulus of nursing and the presence of prolactin.

Breast engorgement with milk is common on days 3–4 postpartum:
- Often painful
- Often accompanied by transient temperature elevation

Suckling stimulates the neurohypophysis to secrete oxytocin in a pulsatile fashion, causing contraction of myoepithelial cells and small milk ducts, leading to milk expression.

Changes in the Blood

- **Leukocytosis** occurs during and after labor (up to 30,000/μL).
- There is a relative **lymphopenia.**
- There is an absolute **eosinopenia.**
- During the first few postpartum days, the **hemoglobin** and **hematocrit** fluctuate moderately from levels just prior to labor.

By 1 week postpartum, the **blood volume** has returned to the patient's non-pregnant range.

CARDIAC OUTPUT

- The **cardiac output** remains elevated for ≥ 48 hours postpartum.
- By 2 weeks postpartum, these changes have returned to nonpregnant levels.

Plasma fibrinogen and the **erythrocyte sedimentation rate** remain for ≥ 1 week postpartum.

Changes in Body Weight

Most women approach their prepregnancy weight 6 months after delivery, but still retain approximately 1.4 kg of excess weight. Five to six kilograms are lost due to uterine evacuation and normal blood loss. Two to three kilograms are lost due to diuresis.

ROUTINE POSTPARTUM CARE

Immediately After Labor

FIRST HOUR

- Take blood pressure (BP) and heart rate (HR) at least every 15 minutes.
- Monitor the amount of vaginal bleeding.

- Palpate the fundus to ensure adequate contraction. If the uterus is relaxed, it should be massaged through the abdominal wall until it remains contracted.

First Several Hours

EARLY AMBULATION

Women are out of bed (OOB) within a few hours after delivery. Advantages include:
- Decreased bladder complications
- Less frequent constipation
- **Reduced frequency of puerperal venous thrombosis and pulmonary embolism**

CARE OF THE VULVA

The patient should be taught to cleanse and wipe the vulva from front to back (toward the anus).

If Episiotomy/Laceration Repair

- An ice pack should be applied for the first several hours to reduce edema and pain.
- At 24 hours postpartum, moist heat (e.g., via warm sitz baths) can decrease local discomfort.
- The episiotomy incision is typically well healed and asymptomatic by week 3 of the puerperium.

BLADDER FUNCTION

Ensure that the postpartum woman has voided within 4 hours of delivery. If not:
- This typically indicates further trouble voiding to follow.
- An indwelling catheter may be necessary, with a prophylactic antibiotic after catheter removal.
- Bladder sensation and capability to empty may be decreased due to anesthesia.
- Consider a hematoma of the genital tract as a possible etiology.

The First Few Days

BOWEL FUNCTION

Lack of a bowel movement may be due to a cleansing enema administered prior to delivery. Encourage early ambulation and feeding to decrease the probability of constipation. Ask the patient about flatus.

If Fourth-Degree Laceration

Fecal incontinence may result, even with correct surgical repair, due to injury to the innervation of the pelvic floor musculature. Keep the patient on a stool softener to avoid straining and decrease risk of fistula formation. Avoid enemas.

Discomfort/Pain Management

During the first few days of the puerperium, pain may result due to:
- Afterpains
- Episiotomy/laceration repair
- Breast engorgement
- Postspinal puncture headache
- Constipation
- Urinary retention

Treat the pain.

Abdominal Wall Relaxation

Exercise may be initiated any time after vaginal delivery and after abdominal discomfort has diminished after cesarean delivery.

Diet

There are *no* dietary restrictions/requirements for women who have delivered vaginally. Two hours postpartum, the mother should be permitted to eat and drink.

Continue iron supplementation for a minimum of 3 months postpartum.

Immunizations

- The nonisoimmunized D-negative mother whose baby is D-positive is given 300 μg of anti-D immune globulin within 72 hours of delivery.
- Mothers not previously immunized against/immune to rubella should be vaccinated prior to discharge.
- Unless contraindicated, mothers may receive a diphtheria–tetanus toxoid booster prior to discharge.

POSTPARTUM PATIENT EDUCATION

The likelihood of significant hemorrhage is greatest immediately postpartum.

Hemostasis is obtained primarily by mechanical clamping of vessels by contracted myometrium.

1. Anticipated physiologic changes during the puerperium:
   - Lochia: The bloody discharge that follows delivery.
   - Diuresis: The secretion and passage of large amounts of urine.
   - Milk letdown: The influx of milk into the mammary ducts.
2. She should go to hospital if she develops:
   - Fever
   - Excessive vaginal bleeding
   - Lower extremity pain and/or swelling
   - Shortness of breath
   - Chest pain
3. Family planning and contraception:
   - Do not wait until first menses to begin contraception; ovulation may come before first menses.
   - Contraception is essential after the first menses, unless a subsequent pregnancy is desired.

Lactational Amenorrhea Method of Contraception

The sole utilization of breast feeding to prevent ovulation and subsequent pregnancy. The lactational amenorrhea method is 98% effective for up to 6 months if:
- The mother is not menstruating.
- The mother is nursing > 2–3 times per night, and ≥ every 4 hours during the day without other supplementation.
- The baby is < 6 months old.

Inadequate postpartum uterine contraction is a major cause of postpartum bleeding.

Combined Oral Contraceptives versus Progestin-Only Contraceptives in Postpartum

Combined oral contraceptive hormones reduce the amount of breast milk, although very small quantities of the hormones are excreted in the milk.

Progestin-only oral contraceptive pills are virtually 100% effective without substantially reducing the amount of breast milk.

Nursing mothers rarely ovulate within the first 10 weeks after delivery. Non-nursing mothers typically ovulate 6–8 weeks after delivery.

Coitus in Postpartum

After 6 weeks, coitus may be resumed based on patient's desire and comfort. A vaginal lubricant prior to coitus may increase comfort.

Dangers of premature intercourse:
- Pain due to continued uterine involution and healing of lacerations/episiotomy scars.
- Increased likelihood of hemorrhage and infection.

Blood can accumulate within the uterus without visible vaginal bleeding: *Watch for:* Palpable uterine **enlargement** during the initial few hours postpartum.

Infant Care

Prior to discharge:
- Follow-up care arrangements should be made.
- All laboratory results should be normal, including:
  - Coombs' test
  - Bilirubin
  - Hemoglobin and hematocrit
  - Blood glucose
- Maternal serologic tests for syphilis and HbsAg should be nonreactive.
- Initial HBV vaccine should be administered.
- All screening tests required by law should be done (e.g., testing for phenylketonuria [PKU] and hypothyroidism).
- Patient education regarding infant immunizations and well-baby care.

Discharge

VAGINAL DELIVERY

One to two days post hospitalization, if no complications.

CESAREAN SECTION

Three to four days post hospitalization, if no complications.

Breast-fed infants are less prone to enteric infections than are bottle-fed babies.

CMV, HBV, and HIV are excreted in breast milk.

A common misperception: Mothers who have a common cold should not breast-feed (FALSE).

Most drugs given to the mother are secreted in breast milk. However, the amount of drug ingested by the infant is typically small.

Breast-Feeding

Human milk is the ideal food for neonates for the first 6 months of life.

RECOMMENDED DIETARY ALLOWANCES

Lactating women need an extra 500 nutritious calories per day. Food choices should be guided by the Food Guide Pyramid, as recommended by the U.S. Department of Health and Human Services/U.S. Department of Agriculture.

BENEFITS

- Uterine involution: Nursing accelerates uterine involution (increases oxytocin).
- Immunity:
  - Colostrum and breast milk contain secretory IgA antibodies against *Escherichia coli* and other potential infections.
  - Milk contains memory T cells, which allows the fetus to benefit from maternal immunologic experience.
  - Colostrum contains interleukin-6, which stimulates an increase in breast milk mononuclear cells.
- Nutrients: All proteins are absorbed by babies, and all essential and nonessential amino acids available.
- Gastrointestinal (GI) maturation: Milk contains epidermal growth factor, which may promote growth and maturation of the intestinal mucosa.

CONTRAINDICATIONS TO BREAST-FEEDING

- **Infection:** Mothers with:
  - Cytomegalovirus (CMV)
  - Chronic hepatitis B (HBV)
  - Human immunodeficiency virus (HIV) infection
  - Breast lesions from active herpes simplex virus
  - Tuberculosis (active, untreated)
- **Medications:** Mothers ingesting the following contraindicated medications (not an exhaustive list):
  - Bromocriptine
  - Cyclophosphamide
  - Cyclosporine
  - Doxorubicin
  - Ergotamine
  - Lithium
  - Methotrexate
- **Drug abuse:** Mothers who abuse the following drugs:
  - Amphetamines
  - Cocaine
  - Heroin
  - Marijuana
  - Nicotine
  - Phencyclidine
  - Ethanol

HIGH-YIELD FACTS

Postpartum

- **Radiotherapy:** Mothers undergoing radiotherapy with:
  - Gallium
  - Indium
  - Iodine
  - Radioactive sodium
  - Technetium

POSTPARTUM PSYCHIATRIC DISORDERS

Maternity/Postpartum Blues

A self-limited, mild mood disturbance due to biochemical factors and psychological stress:
- Affects 50% of women
- Begins within 3–6 days after parturition
- May persist for up to 10 days
- May be related to progesterone withdrawal

SYMPTOMS

Similar to depression, but milder (see below).

TREATMENT

- Supportive—acknowledgment of the mother's feelings and reassurance.
- Monitor for the development of more severe symptoms (i.e., postpartum depression or psychosis).

Postpartum Depression

Similar to minor and major depression that can occur at any time:
- Classified as "postpartum depression" if it begins within 3–6 months after childbirth.
- Eight to fifteen percent of postpartum women develop postpartum depression within 2–3 months.
- Up to 70% recurrence.

SYMPTOMS

Symptoms are the same as major depression.

NATURAL COURSE

- Gradual improvement over the 6-month postpartum period.
- The mother may remain symptomatic for months to years.

TREATMENT

- Pharmacologic intervention is typically required:
  - Antidepressants
  - Anxiolytic agents
  - Electroconvulsive therapy
- Mother should be co-managed with a psychiatrist (i.e., for psychotherapy to focus on any maternal fears or concerns).

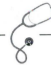

Thirty percent of adolescent women develop postpartum depression.

Criteria for major depression/postpartum depression: Two-week period of depressed mood or anhedonia nearly every day plus one of the following:
1. Significant weight loss or weight gain without effort (or increase or decrease in appetite).
2. Insomnia or hypersomnia.
3. Psychomotor agitation/retardation.
4. Fatigue or loss of energy.
5. Feelings of worthlessness/excessive or inappropriate guilt.
6. Decreased ability to concentrate/think.
7. Recurrent thoughts of suicide/death.

Postpartum Psychosis

- Mothers have an inability to discern reality from that which is unreal (can have periods of lucidity).
- Occurs in 1–4/1,000 births.
- Peak onset—10–14 days postpartum, but may occur months later.

RISK FACTORS

- **History of psychiatric illness**
- **Family history of psychiatric disorders**
- Younger age
- Primiparity

COURSE

Variable and depends on the type of underlying illness; often 6 months.

TREATMENT

- Psychiatric care
- Pharmacologic therapy
- Hospitalization (in most cases)

Medical Conditions and Infections in Pregnancy

Social Risk Factors 98

Contraindications to Pregnancy 100

Nutritional and Physical Activity Recommendations 100

Teratology and Drugs 100

Medical Conditions and Pregnancy 104

Infection and Pregnancy 110

There is no consensus on the quantity of alcohol that leads to adverse fetal outcomes. Hence, the best maternal advice is to discontinue alcohol use when trying to become pregnant and during pregnancy.

Alcohol

- Alcohol is teratogenic (see Table 8-1).
- An occasional drink during pregnancy carries unknown risk.
- Fetal alcohol syndrome (FAS) may occur with chronic exposure to alcohol in the later stages of pregnancy. Features may include:
  - Growth retardation
  - Facial anomalies:
    - Small palpebral fissures
    - Indistinct/absent philtrum
    - Epicanthal folds
    - Flattened nasal bridge
    - Short length of nose
    - Thin upper lip
    - Low-set, unparallel ears
    - Retarded midfacial development
  - Central nervous system (CNS) dysfunction:
    - Microcephaly
    - Mental retardation
    - Abnormal neurobehavior (e.g., attention deficit hyperactivity disorder)

Smoking by pregnant women and all household members should be stopped and not resumed postpartum.

Tobacco

- **The leading preventable cause of low birth weight in the United States** (20–30% of low birth weight in the United States).
- Smoking is associated with decreased birth weight and increased prematurity.
- There is a positive association between smoking and sudden infant death syndrome (SIDS), asthma, chronic respiratory illness, and increased susceptibility to infections.
- Use of nicotine patch is controversial.

Illicit Drugs

MARIJUANA

Derived from the plant *Cannabis sativa*; active ingredient, tetrahydrocannabinol:
- No evidence of significant teratogenesis in humans.
- Metabolites detected in urine of users for days to weeks.
- Commonly used by multiple substance abusers; thus, its presence in urine may identify patients at high risk for being current users of other substances as well and those at risk for sexually transmitted diseases.

COCAINE

- **Resulting complications in pregnancy:**
  - Spontaneous abortion and fetal death in utero, placental abruption
  - Preterm labor and delivery (25%)
  - Meconium-stained amniotic fluid (29%)

- **Teratogenic effects:**
  - Growth retardation
  - Microcephaly
  - Neurobehavioral abnormalities (e.g., impairment in orientation and motor function)
  - SIDS

OPIATES

Heroin

- Three- to sevenfold increase in incidence of stillbirth, fetal growth retardation, prematurity, neonatal mortality, and preeclampsia.
- Signs of infant withdrawal occur 24–72 hours after birth.
- Treatment with methadone improves pregnancy outcome.

Newborn infants born to narcotic addicts are at risk for severe, potentially fatal narcotic withdrawal syndrome, characterized by:
- High-pitched cry
- Poor feeding
- Hypertonicity/tremors
- Irritability
- Sneezing
- Sweating
- Vomiting/diarrhea
- Seizures

HALLUCINOGENS

- No evidence that lysergic acid diethylamide (LSD) or other hallucinogens cause chromosomal damage or other deleterious effects on human pregnancy. However, pregnant women who use LSD very likely engage in other high-risk behaviors that directly harm the fetus.
- There have been no studies on the potential long-term effects on neonatal neurodevelopment.

AMPHETAMINES

Crystal methamphetamine ("ice," "blue ice"), a potent stimulant, is associated with:
- Decreased fetal head circumference
- Placental abruption
- Intrauterine growth retardation (IUGR)
- Fetal death in utero

The anorectic properties of amphetamines can severely impair nutrition during pregnancy.

Exposure to Violence

- **Twenty percent of all pregnant women are battered during pregnancy.**
- **For some women, the violence is initiated at the time of pregnancy.**
- One half of women who are physically abused prior to pregnancy continue to be battered during pregnancy.

- *Ask:* "Are you in a relationship in which you are being hit, kicked, slapped, or threatened?"
- All abused patients should be given information regarding their immediate safety and referrals for counseling and support.

CONTRAINDICATIONS TO PREGNANCY

- **Pulmonary hypertension:** Associated with a 50% maternal mortality rate and a > 40% fetal mortality rate.
- **Eisenmenger syndrome:** Maternal mortality is 30–50%.

NUTRITIONAL AND PHYSICAL ACTIVITY RECOMMENDATIONS

Nutritional Recommendations

Folic acid supplementation reduces the risk of NTDs.

- Folic acid supplementation:
  - If pregnancy is high risk for neural tube defect (NTD): 4 mg/day starting 4 weeks prior to conception, through the first trimester.
  - 0.4 mg (400 μg) daily for all women planning on pregnancy.

Physical Activity Recommendations

The neural tube is nearly formed by the time of the first missed period. Starting folic acid supplementation when pregnancy is diagnosed is too late.

- Women who exercise regularly before pregnancy are encouraged to continue.
- For the normal healthy woman, a low-impact exercise regimen may be continued throughout pregnancy.

TERATOLOGY AND DRUGS

The placenta permits the passage of many drugs and dietary substances (see Table 8-1):

Drug exposure is responsible for 2–3% of birth defects.

- Lipid-soluble substances readily cross the placenta.
- Water-soluble substances cross less well because of their larger molecular weight.
- The greater degree to which a drug is bound to plasma protein, the less likely it is free to cross.
- **The minimal effective dose (for any drug) should be employed.**

Embryological Age and Teratogenic Susceptibility

- 0–3 weeks—**predifferentiation phase of development:** The conceptus either does not survive exposure to teratogen or survives without anomalies.
- 3–8 weeks—**organogenesis phase:** Maximum susceptibility to teratogen-induced malformation.
- > 8 weeks—**organ growth phase:** A teratogen can interfere with growth but not organogenesis.

TABLE 8-1. Common Teratogenic Substances

Substance	Fetal Effects
ACE inhibitors	Renal defects, neonatal renal failure, lack of cranial ossification, and growth restriction. Worst effects in second- or third-trimester exposure.
Alcohol	Pre- and postnatal growth restriction, mental retardation, microcephaly, midfacial hypoplasia, renal and cardiac defects, FAS. (*Note:* The risk of one to two drinks daily is unknown; therefore, ingestion of alcohol, even at low levels, is generally not advised in pregnancy.)
Aminoglycosides	Hearing loss, eighth cranial nerve damage, renal defects. (*Note:* Effects are commonly associated with streptomycin and tobramycin; other agents in class may be safe.)
Anabolic steroids, synthetic testosterone analogs (e.g., Danazol)	Masculinization (virilization) of females, advanced genital formation in males.
Antineoplastics	Many.
Benzodiazepines	Were thought to be associated with cleft lip/palate, especially diazepam; newer studies dispute this.
Carbamazepine	Craniofacial and CNS defects, NTDs, microcephaly, growth restriction, fingernail hypoplasia.
Cocaine	Bowel atresia, cardiac defects, cerebral infarcts, mental retardation, growth restriction.
Coumadin	Craniofacial and CNS defects, growth restriction, spontaneous abortion or stillbirth.
DHT synthesis inhibitors (e.g., finasteride)	Feminization of males.
DES	Vaginal or cervical clear cell adenocarcinoma, vaginal adenosis, cervical incompetence, infertility.
Folic acid antagonists (e.g., aminopterin, methotrexate)	Nervous system defects, cleft lip/palate, growth restriction, increased risk of spontaneous abortion.
Iodine	Goiter, cretinism
Lead	Increased rate of spontaneous abortion and stillbirth.
Lithium	Ebstein's anomaly and other cardiac defects.
Mercury (organic)	Cerebral atrophy, microcephaly, mental retardation, cerebral palsy, blindness. Exposure generally associated with consumption of fish or grain contaminated with methyl mercury.

HIGH-YIELD FACTS

Conditions and Infections

TABLE 8-1. Common Teratogenic Substances (continued)

SUBSTANCE	FETAL EFFECTS
Phenytoin	Cardiovascular and nervous system defects, mental retardation, microcephaly, craniofacial and limb defects, growth restriction.
Radiation	Microcephaly, mental retardation, leukemia.
Tetracycline	Yellow or brown teeth if exposed in second or third trimester.
Thalidomide	Phocomelia, cardiac and gastrointestinal defects. Worst (20% rate) if between 35 and 50 days' gestation.
Tobacco	Growth restriction, low birth weight, prematurity.
Trimethadione, paramethadione	Craniofacial and cardiac defects, microcephaly, growth restriction, mental retardation.
Valproic acid	NTDs (especially spina bifida), hypospadias. First-trimester exposure is the most dangerous.
Vitamin A derivatives (e.g., isotretinoin, tretinoin, etretinate)	Craniofacial and cardiac defects, nervous system defects, thymic agenesis, mental retardation, increased rate of spontaneous abortion.

ACE, angiotensin-converting enzyme; CNS, central nervous system; DES, diethylstilbestrol; DHT, dihydrotestosterone; FAS, fetal alcohol syndrome; NTD, neural tube defect.

FDA (Food and Drug Administration) Pregnancy Drug Categories

See Table 8-2.

Anticoagulants

- Warfarin (Coumadin) crosses the placenta and is associated with chondrodysplasia punctata, presumably due to microhemorrhages during development (nasal hypoplasia).
  - Fetal and maternal hemorrhage has also been reported, but incidence can be reduced with careful control of the prothrombin time.
- Heparin, an alternative to Coumadin, has a large negative charge and does *not* cross the placenta.
  - Does *not* have any adverse fetal effects.
  - Heparin-induced osteoporosis with fracture occurs in 1–2% of women in whom full anticoagulation has been achieved during pregnancy.
- Low-molecular-weight heparin (LMWH):
  - May have substantial benefit over standard unfractionated heparin.
  - Molecules do *not* cross placenta.

Warfarin exposure:
1/6 abnormal liveborn
1/6 abortion/stillbirth

Heparin is the drug of choice in pregnant patients who require anticoagulation.

TABLE 8-2. Food and Drug Administration Drug Categories

CATEGORY	MEANING
A	Safety has been established using human studies.
B	Presumed safety based on animal studies.
C	Uncertain safety—animal studies show an adverse effect, no human studies.
D	Unsafe—proven evidence of risk; use may be justifiable in certain clinical situations.
X	Highly unsafe—proven evidence of risk that outweighs any possible benefit.

Hypoglycemic Agents

Insulin is safe in pregnancy:
- Does *not* cross the placenta per large molecular weight (6,000).
- Dosage is unimportant as long as it is sufficient to maintain normal maternal glucose levels.

Glyburide is an alternative to insulin.

Low-molecular-weight heparin may be used in pregnancy.

Psychotropics

ANTIDEPRESSANTS

- Imipramine (Tofranil): Tricyclic antidepressant; associated with fetal cardiac anomalies.
- Fluoxetine (Paxil): No increased risk of major malformations or developmental abnormalities have been observed.

TRANQUILIZERS

- Chlordiazepoxide (Librium) is associated with congenital anomalies.
- Diazepam use perinatally has been associated with fetal hypothermia, hypotonia, and respiratory depression.

Analgesics

- Aspirin:
  - No teratogenic effects seen in T1.
  - Significant perinatal effects seen, such as decreased uterine contractility, delayed onset of labor, prolonged duration of labor.
  - Increases risk of antepartum bleeding and bleeding at delivery.
- Nonsteroidal anti-inflammatory drugs (NSAIDs):
  - Ibuprofen (Motrin, Advil) and naproxen (Naprosyn) have not demonstrated any negative fetal effects with short-term use.
  - Chronic use may lead to oligohydramnios and constriction of the fetal ductus arteriosus.

Nonpharmacologic remedies such as rest and local heat should be recommended for aches and pains if possible before analgesics.

Pregnant patients are susceptible to vaginal yeast infections; hence, antibiotics should be used only when clearly indicated.

■ Acetaminophen (Tylenol, Datril) has shown no evidence of teratogenicity.

Antibiotics and Anti-infective Agents

■ Penicillins, cephalosporins, and erythromycin are safe in pregnancy.
■ Trimethoprim use in T1 is associated with increased risk of birth defects.
■ Doxycycline has no teratogenic risk in T1.
■ Quinolones (ciprofloxacin, norfloxacin) have a high affinity for cartilage and bone tissue and may cause arthropathies in children.

Antiasthmatics

■ Epinephrine (sympathomimetic amine) exposure after T1 has been associated with minor malformations.
■ Terbutaline (Brethine) is not associated with birth defects. Long-term use has been associated with increased risk of glucose intolerance.
■ Isoproterenol (Isuprel) and albuterol (Ventolin) are not teratogenic.
■ Corticosteroids are inactivated by the placenta when maternally administered; < 10% of maternal dose is in the fetus.

Cardiovascular Drugs

■ Propranolol (Inderal) shows no evidence of teratogenicity:
  ■ Fetal bradycardia has been seen as a direct dose effect when given to mother 2 hours prior to delivery.
  ■ Increased risk of IUGR seen with maternal use.

MEDICAL CONDITIONS AND PREGNANCY

Endocrine Disorders in Pregnancy

DIABETES MELLITUS

Pregnancy testing is recommended before prescribing hormonal medications in patients with anovulatory symptoms and menstrual irregularities.

■ **Pregestational diabetes (DM)**—patient had DM before pregnancy.
■ **Gestational diabetes (GDM)**—patient develops diabetes only during pregnancy.
  ■ White classification A1—controlled with diet
  ■ White classification A2—requires insulin

Screening

Screening is controversial, but tests often used are:

1. **Glucose challenge test**—at 26–28 weeks:
   ■ Give 50g glucose load (nonfasting state).
   ■ Draw glucose blood level 1 hour later.
   ■ > 140 is high (a 3-hour glucose tolerance test is then required to diagnose GDM).
   ■ If ≥ 200, patient is diagnosed with GDM type A1 and a diabetic diet is initiated.

2. **3-hour glucose tolerance test**—if glucose challenge test is > 140 and < 200:
   - Draw fasting glucose level; normal (n) < 95.
   - Give 100g glucose load.
   - Draw glucose levels at 1 hour (n < 180), at 2 hours (n < 155), and at 3 hours (n < 140).
   - Positive for gestational diabetes if 2/4 high values.

Diabetes is the most common medical complication of pregnancy.

Risk Factors

- **Be extra careful to test:**
  - Age > 25
  - Previous or family history of gestational diabetes
  - Obesity
  - History of large babies
  - History of full-term stillbirth or child with cardiac defects (poor obstetrical outcome)
  - Race: Black, Hispanic, Native American

Gestational diabetes probably results from **placental lactogen** secreted during pregnancy, which has large glucagon-like effects.

Effects of Gestational Diabetes

Maternal Effects
- Four times increased risk of preeclampsia
- Increased risk of bacterial infections
- Higher rate of C-section
- Increased risk of polyhydramnios
- Increased risk of birth injury

Fetal Effects
- Increased risk of perinatal death
- Three times increased risk of fetal anomalies (renal, cardiac, and CNS)
- Two to three times increased risk of preterm delivery
- Fetal macrosomia increases risk of birth injury
- Metabolic derangements (hypoglycemia, hypocalcemia)

Thirty percent of women with gestational diabetes develop other diabetes later.

Management

The key factors involved in successful management of these high-risk pregnancies include:
- Good glucose control:
  - Prepregnancy glucose levels should be maintained during pregnancy with insulin.
  - Glucose control should be checked at each prenatal visit.

The CNS anomaly most specific to DM is **caudal regression.**

Starting at 32–34 Weeks
- **Fetal monitoring:**
  - Ultrasonography to evaluate fetal growth, estimated weight, amniotic fluid volume, and fetal anatomy.
  - Nonstress test and amniotic fluid index testing weekly to biweekly depending on disease severity.
  - Biophysical profile.
  - Contraction stress test (oxytocin challenge test).
- **Early elective delivery:**
  - Fetal macrosomia must be ruled out with ultrasonography.

In normal pregnancy, total T_3, T_4, and thyroid-binding globulin (TBG) are elevated, but free thyroxine levels do not change = euthyroid.

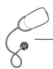

Propylthiouracil (PTU) is the drug of choice over methimazole for treating thyrotoxicosis in pregnancy.

Overt hypothyroidism is often associated with infertility.

In women with type 1 DM, 25% develop postpartum thyroid dysfunction.

Folic acid supplementation is increased in the epileptic patient to 5 mg/day.

- If fetal weight is > 4,500 g, elective cesarean section should be considered to avoid shoulder dystocia. Unless there is an obstetric complication, induction of labor and vaginal delivery are done.

THYROID AND PITUITARY DISEASE

Thyrotoxicosis/Thyroid Storm

- Twenty-five percent mortality rate.
- Thyrotoxicosis complicates 1/2,000 pregnancies.
- Graves' disease is the most common cause of thyrotoxicosis in pregnancy.
- Precipitating factors are infection, labor, and C-section.
- Treatment is propylthiouricil or methimazole or surgery. **Radioactive iodine is contraindicated in pregnancy.**

Treatment
- β blocker
- Sodium iodide
- Parathyroid hormone (PTH)
- Dexamethasone

Complications
- 1% risk of neonatal thyrotoxicosis
- Fetal goiter/hypothyroid, usually from propylthiouracil
- Preterm delivery
- Preeclampsia
- Preterm delivery

Hypothyroidism

Subclinical hypothyroidism is more common than overt hypothyroidism, and often goes unnoticed. Diagnosed by elevated TSH.

Postpartum Thyroiditis

Transient postpartum hypothyroidism or thyrotoxicosis associated with autoimmune thyroiditis is common:
- Between 1 and 4 months postpartum, 4% of all women develop transient thyrotoxicosis.
- Between 4 and 8 months postpartum, 2–5% of all women develop hypothyroidism.

Sheehan Syndrome

Pituitary ischemia and necrosis associated with obstetrical blood loss leading to hypopituitarism. Patients do not lactate postpartum due to low prolactin.

Epilepsy and Pregnancy

- Epileptic women taking anticonvulsants during pregnancy have double the general population risk of malformations and preeclampsia.
- Women with a convulsive disorder have an increased risk of birth defects even when they do not take anticonvulsant medications.
- Pregnant epileptics are more prone to seizures due to the associated stress and fatigue of pregnancy.

- The fetus is at risk for megaloblastic anemia.
- The pregnant female and her fetus are at risk for hemorrhage due to a deficiency of vitamin K–dependent clotting factors induced by anticonvulsant drugs.
- Management of the epileptic female should begin with prepregnancy counseling.
- Anticonvulsant therapy should be reduced to the minimum dose of the minimum number of anticonvulsant medications.
- Folic acid supplementation (5 mg/day) should be taken by those women taking anticonvulsants.
- Once pregnant, the patient should be screened for NTDs and congenital malformations.
- Blood levels of anticonvulsant medications should be checked at the beginning of pregnancy to determine the drug level that controls epileptic episodes successfully.

HIV and Pregnancy

At the preconception visit, encourage maternal HIV screening.

- HIV infection is now among the 10 leading causes of death among children aged 1–4 years.
- The vast majority of cases of pediatric AIDS are secondary to vertical transmission from mother to fetus.

THE HIV-POSITIVE PATIENT

- Reduce maternal viral load.
  - Zidovudine (ZDV) should be given in the antepartum period beginning at 14 weeks.
  - CD4+ counts and viral loads should be monitored at regular intervals.
  - Blood counts and liver functions should be monitored monthly while patient is on ZDV.
- Reduce vertical transmission.
  - Give maternal intravenous ZDV.
  - Reduce duration of ruptured membranes.
  - Offer elective C-section to mother.
  - Avoid breast-feeding.
- Administer newborn prophylaxis.
  - Give ZDV syrup to newborn for 6 weeks.

Cardiovascular Disease

- Pregnancy-induced hemodynamic changes have profound effects on underlying heart disease.
- **Cardiovascular disease (CVD) complicates 1% of all pregnancies and significantly contributes to maternal mortality.**

MITRAL STENOSIS (MS)

Pathophysiology

Increased preload due to normal increase in blood volume results in left atrial overload and backup into the lungs resulting in **pulmonary hypertension.**

Combination ZDV and C-section decreases vertical transmission of HIV by up to 85%.

The majority of new cases of AIDS in women are among those 20–29 years of age.

Rate of perinatal HIV transmission ≈ 30%.

Anemia commonly occurs in mothers on ZDV.

Cardiac output increases by 30–50% by midpregnancy.

Blood volume increases 50% by 30th week.

Twenty-five percent of women with mitral stenosis have cardiac failure for the first time during pregnancy.

Prolapse = okay to be Pregnant
Stenosis = Sick in pregnancy

Asthmatics have a small but significant increase in pregnancy complications.

Pregnancy is a hypercoagulable state.

Half of patients with asymptomatic deep venous thrombosis have PEs.

Sequelae

- Tachycardia associated with labor and delivery exacerbates the pulmonary HTN because of decreased filling time. May lead to pulmonary edema.
- **Peripartum period is the most hazardous time.**

Treatment

Antibiotic prophylaxis.

MITRAL VALVE PROLAPSE

These patients are normally asymptomatic and have a systolic click on physical exam. They will generally have a safe pregnancy. Antibiotics should be give for prophylaxis against endocarditis.

EISENMENGER SYNDROME AND OTHER CONDITIONS WITH PULMONARY HTN

These conditions are extremely dangerous to the mother and possibly justify the termination of pregnancies on medical grounds. Maternal mortality can be as high as 50%, with death usually occurring postpartum.

AORTIC STENOSIS

- Similar problems with mitral stenosis.
- Avoid tachycardia and fluid overload.
- Give antibiotic prophylaxis.

Pulmonary Disease

The adaptations to the respiratory system during pregnancy must be able to satisfy the increased O_2 demands of the hyperdynamic circulation and the fetus. Advanced pregnancy may worsen the pathophysiological effects of many acute and chronic lung diseases.

ASTHMA

Epidemiology

One to four percent of pregnancies are complicated by asthma:
- 25% of asthmatics worsen in pregnancy.
- 25% improve.
- 50% have no change.

Management

- Generally, asthma is exacerbated by respiratory tract infections, so killed influenza vaccine should be given.
- Pregnant asthmatics can be treated with β agonists, epinephrine, and steroids (the usual medications).

PULMONARY EMBOLISM (PE)

The likelihood of venous thromboembolism in normal pregnancy and the puerperium is increased fivefold when compared to nonpregnant women of similar age:
- Occurs in 1/7,000 women.

- Complications include maternal death.
- Start anticoagulation with heparin/LMWH.

Renal and Urinary Tract Disorders

Pregnancy causes hydronephrosis (dilatation of renal pelvis, calyces, and ureters) because the baby compresses the lower ureter and because the hormonal milieu decreases ureteral tone. This may lead to urinary stasis and increased vesicoureteral reflux.

Two to seven percent of pregnant women have urinary tract infections (UTIs); 25% are asymptomatic.

PYELONEPHRITIS

Acute pyelonephritis is the most common serious medical complication of pregnancy and occurs in 1–2% of pregnant women. Management includes:
- Hospitalization
- IV antibiotics (ampicillin or cefazolin)
- Monitor fluids
- Decreased incidence with treatment of asymptomatic bacteriuria

Acute Abdomen in Pregnancy

During advanced pregnancy, GI symptoms become difficult to assess and physical findings are often obscured by the enlarged uterus.

Differential
- Pylonephritis
- Appendicitis
- Pancreatitis
- Cholecystitis
- Ovarian torsion
- Ectopic pregnancy (early pregnancy)
- Labor

APPENDICITIS

- Appendicitis is the most common surgical condition in pregnancy (occurs 1/2,000 births).
- Has usual symptoms.
- Uterus displaces the appendix superiorly and laterally. Pain and tenderness may not be found at McBurney's point (RLQ).
- May be difficult to diagnose.
- Physical exam likely to be obscured due to enlarging uterus.
- Incidence is same throughout pregnancy, but rupture is more frequent in T3 (40%) than T1 (10%).
- Management is appendectomy.

CHOLELITHIASIS AND CHOLECYSTITIS

- Incidence of cholecystitis is 1/1,000 pregnancies (more common than nonpregnant).
- Same clinical picture as nonpregnant.
- Medical management unless common bile duct obstruction or pancreatitis develops, in which case a cholescystectomy should be perfomed.
- High risk of preterm labor.

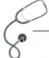

Dangers of appendix rupture:
- Abortion
- Preterm labor
- Maternal–fetal sepsis → neonatal neurologic injury

Remember, there may be physiologic leukocytosis during pregnancy.

Increased estrogens cause **increase in cholesterol** saturation, which, in addition to **biliary stasis**, leads to **more gallstones** in pregnant women.

Persistent nausea and vomiting in *late* pregnancy should prompt a search for underlying pathology (e.g., gastroenteritis, cholecystitis, pancreatitis, hepatitis, peptic ulcer, pyelonephritis, fatty liver of pregnancy, and psychological or social issues).

The two most common causes of anemia during pregnancy and the puerperium are iron deficiency and acute blood loss.

Anemia

- *Physiologic anemia* is normal anemia in pregnancy because of hemodilution due to volume expansion.
- Anemia for a pregnant woman is a drop in hemoglobin below 10 g/dL or hematocrit < 30%.
- **Incidence:** 20–60% of pregnant women, 80% is iron-deficiency type.
- **Risks:** Preterm delivery, IUGR, low birth weight.
- Therapy is 325 mg tid of $FeSO_4$.

INFECTION AND PREGNANCY

See Tables 8-2 through 8-4.

Toxoplasma
Other (syphilis, HIV, parvovirus)
Rubella
Cytomegalovirus
Herpes

TABLE 8-2. Perinatal Infections

INTRAUTERINE[a]	VIRAL	BACTERIAL	PROTOZOAN
Transplacental	Varicella-zoster	*Listeria*	Toxoplasmosis
	Coxsackie virus	Syphilis	Malaria
	Parvovirus		
	Rubella		
	Cytomegalovirus		
	HIV		
	Hepatitis		
Ascending infection	HSV	GBS	
		Coliforms, GC/chlamydia	
INTRAPARTUM[b]			
Maternal exposure	HSV	Gonorrhea	
	Papillomavirus	*Chlamydia*	
	HIV	GBS	
	HBV	TB	
External contamination	HSV	*Staphylococcus*	
		Coliforms	
NEONATAL			
Human transmission	HSV	*Staphylococcus*	
Respirators and catheters		*Staphylococcus*	
		Coliforms	

[a] Bacteria, viruses, or parasites may gain access transplacentally or cross the intact membranes.
[b] Organisms may colonize and infect the fetus during L&D.
GBS, group B Streptococcus; GC, gonococcus; HBV, hepatitis B virus; HIV, human immunodeficiency virus; HSV, herpes simplex virus; TB, tuberculosis.

TABLE 8-3. Viral Infections and Their Potential Fetal Effects

Virus	Fetal Effects	Maternal Effects	Prophylaxis	Treatment
Varicella-zoster[a]	**Transmitted transplacentally** ■ Chorioretinitis ■ Cerebral cortical atrophy ■ Hydronephrosis ■ Cutaneous and bony leg defects (scars) ■ Microcephaly	Pneumonitis Chickenpox	Vaccine *not* recommended for pregnant women.	Varicella-zoster immunoglobulin within 96 hrs of exposure. C-section should be performed if there are active lesions.
Orthomyxoviridae (influenza)	■ Neural tube defects	■ Pneumonia ■ Flu ■ Death	Vaccination is recommended for pregnant women who have chronic underlying disease or who are routinely exposed.	Amantadine within 48 hrs of onset of symptoms in non-immunized, high-risk patients.
Parvovirus B19	■ Abortion ■ Death ■ Congenital anomalies ■ Hydrops	Viremia → slapped cheek appearance		If + serology → US; if + hydrops → consider fetal transfusion.
Rubella	**Congenital rubella syndrome** ■ Anemia ■ Cataracts/glaucoma ■ Patent ductus arteriosus ■ Deafness ■ Mental retardation		Vaccination (attenuated live virus) of the non-pregnant female.	Consider therapeutic abortion, depending on time of exposure during pregnancy.
Hepatitis B		Range from mild liver dysfunction to death	Maternal screening early in pregnancy. Maternal HBsAg positive is high risk of transmitting to fetus. If mother is positive, give neonate HepB IgG at birth, 3 months, and 6 months.	

HIGH-YIELD FACTS

Conditions and Infections

VIRUS	FETAL EFFECTS	MATERNAL EFFECTS	PROPHYLAXIS	TREATMENT
Cytomegalovirus	Causes in utero infection in 1% of all newborns but only 10% of infected show disease. ■ **Cytomegalic inclusion disease** 　■ Hepatospleno-megaly 　■ Thrombocytopenia 　■ Microcephaly 　■ Intracranial calcifications 　■ Chorioretinitis 　■ Mental retardation 　■ Jaundice	Mononucleosis-like syndrome		None.

a Infection may be especially severe in pregnant women.

TABLE 8-4. Bacterial Infections and Their Potential Fetal Effects

BACTERIA	FETAL EFFECTS	MATERNAL EFFECTS	PROPHYLAXIS	TREATMENT
Group B *Streptococcus* (*Streptococcus agalactiae*)	■ Preterm labor ■ Premature rupture of membranes ■ Ophthalmia neonatorum ■ Sepsis ■ Meningitis → neurologic sequelae in survivors	■ Chorioamnionitis ■ Puerperal sepsis ■ Mastitis ■ Osteomyelitis	Intrapartum maternal penicillin G in women with + cultures at 35–37 wks' GA or high risk	Neonatal penicillin G IM in the delivery room (there is no universal treatment)
Salmonella	■ Death	■ Enteritis ■ Bacteremia		IV fluid rehydration*a*
Borrelia burgdorferi (Lyme)	■ Congenital infection ■ Death ■ Preterm labor ■ Rash	■ Erythema migrans ■ Disseminated infection ■ Meningitis ■ Carditis ■ Arthritis		Oral amoxicillin or penicillin

BACTERIA	FETAL EFFECTS	MATERNAL EFFECTS	PROPHYLAXIS	TREATMENT
Primary and secondary syphilis	■ Hepatosplenomegaly ■ Lymphadenopathy ■ Hemolysis			
Chlamydia trachomatis	■ Conjunctivitis ■ Pneumonia		Screen in early pregnancy	Erythromycin or azithromycin
Neisseria gonorrhoeae	■ Conjunctivitis ■ Otitis externa ■ Pharyngitis		Screen in early pregnancy	Penicillin or ceftriaxone

Toxoplasma gondii	Transplacental infection occurs.
	■ Congenital disease
	  ■ Hydrocephaly/ microcephaly
	  ■ Hepatospleno-megaly
	  ■ Seizures
	  ■ Intracranial calcifications
	  ■ Chorioretinitis
	  ■ Mental retardation
				Spiramycin (macrolide antibiotic)

a Antimicrobials prolong the carrier state and are not given in uncomplicated infections.

Complications of Pregnancy

Hypertension in Pregnancy	116
Preterm Labor	119
Premature Rupture of Membranes	123
Third-Trimester Bleeding	125
Abnormalities of the Third Stage of Labor	130
Postpartum Infection	133

Hypertensive Diseases of Pregnancy

These include transient hypertension, chronic hypertension during pregnancy, and preeclampsia.

There are four categories of hypertension in pregnancy:

1. **Transient hypertension** (most benign):
   - A sustained or transient systolic BP ≥ 140 mm Hg and/or diastolic BP ≥ 90 mm Hg occurs after the 20th week of gestation without proteinuria or end-organ damage.
   - Patient was normotensive prior to and during early pregnancy and become hypertensive late in pregnancy, during labor, or ≤ 24 hours postpartum.
   - By definition, blood pressure must return to normal within 10 days after giving birth.
2. **Preexisting or chronic hypertension during pregnancy:**
   - In preexisting hypertension, the hypertension begins prior to pregnancy.
   - In chronic hypertension during pregnancy, a sustained systolic BP ≥ 140 mm Hg and/or diastolic BP ≥ 90 mm Hg occurs *prior* to the 20th week of gestation.
   - Neither is associated with significant proteinuria or end-organ damage, and both persist after delivery.
3. **Preeclampsia:**
   - Defined as proteinuria and edema in the setting of hypertension after the 20th week of gestation.
   - Mild preeclampsia is defined by:
     - A systolic BP ≥ 140 mm Hg or a diastolic BP ≥ 90 mm Hg on two occasions > 6 hours apart.
     - Proteinuria (> 300 mg/24 hrs)
   - Severe preeclampsia is defined by:
     - A systolic BP ≥ 160 mm Hg or a diastolic BP ≥ 110 mm Hg.
     - Significant proteinuria (≥ 5.0 g/day).
     - Evidence of end-organ damage (e.g., visual disturbances, headache, hyperreflexia, confusion, abdominal pain, impaired liver function/hyperbilirubinemia, pulmonary edema, microangiopathic hemolytic anemia or thrombocytopenia).
4. **Preeclampsia (mild or severe) in patients with preexisting hypertension or with chronic hypertension in pregnancy.**
   - Patients can have hypertension prior to pregnancy and develop preeclampsia.
   - Patients can have seemingly benign hypertension (no proteinuria or evidence of end-organ damage) occurring during early pregnancy and develop preeclampsia.
   - Proteinuria and edema in the setting of hypertension after the 20th week of gestation is preeclampsia, regardless of the timing of the onset of the hypertension.

Pathophysiology

- Preeclampsia: Believed to be caused by reduced placental perfusion leading to a release of factors that:

The only cure for hypertension in pregnancy (except preexisting chronic hypertension) is delivery.

Hypertension-related deaths in pregnancy account for 15% (second after pulmonary embolism) of maternal deaths.

In pregnancy-induced hypertension (PIH), you must monitor for intrauterine growth retardation (IUGR) and progression to superimposed preeclampsia (15–25% incidence).

Severe PIH usually occurs in the third trimester.

Complications of Pregnancy

- Increase vascular responsiveness to vasoconstrictors.
- Activate the coagulation cascade.
- Transient hypertension/chronic hypertension in pregnancy:
  - Unknown.
  - May indicate increased risk of chronic hypertension later in life.

Treatment

See Figure 9-1 for a management algorithm.

- Preexisting hypertension/transient hypertension/chronic hypertension in pregnancy: Antihypertensive medications vs. close observation.
- Mild preeclampsia:
  - Vitamins C and E and calcium supplementation have all been thought to be prophylactic for preeclampsia, but recent studies suggest otherwise.
  - Prompt delivery if mature infant (≥ 34 weeks' gestation) or if fetal lung maturity has been documented by amniocentesis.
  - Close and frequent follow-up.
  - Bed rest.
  - Seizure precautions.
  - Antihypertensive medications.
- Severe preeclampsia:
  - Hospitalization.
  - Close monitoring.
  - If deteriorating or deterioration imminent: Consider prompt delivery regardless of fetal age/maturity.
  - Start MgSo$_4$ for seizure prophylaxis.

HELLP Syndrome

HELLP syndrome is a manifestation of severe preeclampsia with **H**emolysis, **E**levated **L**iver enzymes, and **L**ow **P**latelets. In contrast to typical presentations of preeclampsia, it is associated with:
- High morbidity
- Multiparous mothers
- Mothers older than 25
- Less than 37 weeks' gestation (80%)

Eclampsia

Defined as seizure or coma without another cause in a patient with preeclampsia.

Treatment

- Rule out other causes: Head trauma is a possible confounder; others include cerebral tumors, cerebral venous thrombosis, drug overdoses, epilepsy, or cerebrovascular accidents.
- Delivery is the only definitive treatment. Emergent C-section once seizures abate and patient is stabilized.
- Airway, breathing, and circulation (ABCs).
- Correct hypoxia and acidosis.
- Control seizures with magnesium sulfate (the only anticonvulsant used).
- Control BP with hydralazine or labetalol.

Symptoms of severe disease include:
- Headache
- Visual disturbances
- Epigastric pain

The only definitive treatment for PIH is delivery.

Preeclampsia is usually asymptomatic; it is crucial to pick up during routine prenatal visits.

Hypertension may be absent in 20% of women with HELLP syndrome and severe in 50%.

The relationship between HELLP syndrome and preeclampsia is controversial.

The prime objectives in the management of severe preeclampsia are to forestall convulsions, prevent intracranial hemorrhage and serious damage to other vital organs, and deliver a healthy infant.

Diuretics are not used in pregnancy because they decrease plasma volume and this may be detrimental to fetal growth. Salt restriction also decreases plasma volume and is not recommended.

Angiotensin-converting enzyme (ACE) inhibitors are contraindicated because they are teratogenic. Use other classes of antihypertensives to control hypertension in pregnancy.

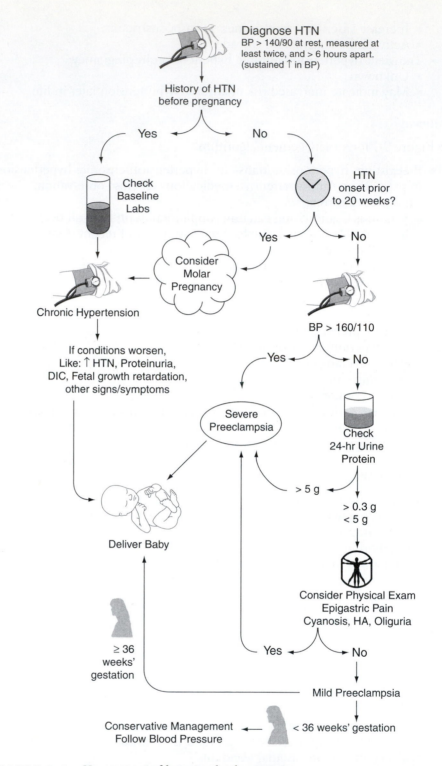

FIGURE 9-1. Management of hypertension in pregnancy.

(Redrawn, with permission, from Lindarkis NM, Lott S. *Digging Up the Bones: Obstetrics and Gynecology.* New York: McGraw-Hill, 1998: 60.)

ANTIHYPERTENSIVE AGENTS USED IN PREGNANCY

Short-Term Control

- *Hydralazine:* IV or PO, direct vasodilator
  Side effects: Systemic lupus erythematosus (SLE)-like syndrome, headache, palpitations
- *Labetalol:* IV or PO, nonselective β_1 and α_1 blocker
  Side effects: Headache and tremor

Long-Term Control

- *Methyldopa:* PO, false neurotransmitter
  Side effects: Postural hypotension, drowsiness, fluid retention
- *Nifedipine:* PO, calcium channel blocker
  Side effects: Edema, dizziness
- *Atenolol:* PO, selective β_1 blocker
  Side effect: breathlessness

SEIZURES IN ECLAMPSIA
- 25% of seizures are before labor.
- 50% of seizures are during labor.
- 25% of seizures are post-labor (may be encountered up to 10 days postpartum).

PRETERM LABOR

Risk

Admission to the hospital in apparent labor prior to the 37th week of gestation. A system has been developed to predict the risk of preterm labor (see Table 9-1).

Criteria

Gestational age (GA) < 37 weeks with regular uterine contractions and:
- Progressive cervical change
  or
- A cervix that is 2 cm dilated
  or
- A cervix 80% effaced
  or
- Ruptured membranes

Magnesium toxicity (7 to 10 mEq/L) is associated with loss of patellar reflexes. Treat with calcium gluconate 10% solution 1 g IV.

Assessment

- Frequency of uterine contractions.
- Possible causes such as infection, abruption.
- Confirm GA of fetus (i.e., by ultrasound).
- Assess fetal well-being with a biophysical profile.

Management of Preterm Labor

Hydration
Not proven to reduce preterm labor, but always hydrate first. May stop contractions. Dehydration causes antidiuretic hormone (ADH) secretion, and ADH mimics oxytocin, which causes uterine contractions.

Tocolytic Therapy
Tocolysis is the pharmacologic inhibition of uterine contractions. It is used if < 34 weeks' gestation.

Braxton Hicks contractions (irregular, nonrhythmical, usually painless contractions that begin at early gestation and increase as term approaches) may make it difficult to distinguish between true and false labor.

Complications of Pregnancy

Most infants born after 34 weeks' GA will survive (the survival rate is within 1% of the survival rate beyond 37 weeks).

TABLE 9-1. Preterm Labor Risk

PARAMETER	FINDING	POINTS
Age of the patient	< 18 years of age	4
	18 or 19 years of age	2
	20–40 years of age	0
	> 40 years of age	2
Height	< 150 cm	3
	≥ 150 cm	0
Weight	< 45 kg	3
	≥ 45 kg	0
Socioeconomic status	Very low	3
	Low	1
	Middle to upper class	0
Single parent	Yes	2
	No	0
Number of children at home	2 (assume ≥ 2)	1
	0 or 1	0
Number of abortions	0	0
	1	1
	2	2
	3 (assume ≥ 3)	3
Length of time since last pregnancy	< 1 year	1
	≥ 1 year	0
History of pyelonephritis	No	0
	Yes	4
Uterine anomaly	Absent	0
	Present	5
History of diethylstilbestrol (DES) exposure	No	0
	Yes	5
History of premature delivery	No	0
	Yes	10
History of second-trimester abortion	No	0
	Single	5
	Repeated	10
Work location	At home	0
	Outside home	1

TABLE 9-1. Preterm Labor Risk (continued)

PARAMETER	FINDING	POINTS
Intensity of work	Light to moderate	0
	Heavy	3
Smoking	> 10 cigarettes per day	2
	≤ 10 cigarettes per day	0
Travel	Long and tiring	3
	Not long and tiring	0
Unusual fatigue during current pregnancy	Present	1
	Absent	0
Weight gain by 32 weeks during current pregnancy	< 13 kg	2
	≥ 13 kg	0
Albuminuria during current pregnancy	Absent	0
	Present	2
Hypertension during current pregnancy	Present	2
	Absent	0
Bacteriuria during current pregnancy	Present	2
	Absent	0
Breech at 32 weeks	Absent	0
	Present	3
Weight loss	< 2 kg	0
	≥ 2 kg	3
Head engaged during current pregnancy	Present	3
	Absent	0
Febrile illness during current pregnancy	Present	3
	Absent	0
Metrorrhagia after 12 weeks' gestation	Present	4
	Absent	0
Effacement	Present	4
	Absent	0
Cervical dilatation	Present	4
	Absent	0
Uterine irritability	Present	4
	Absent	0

TABLE 9-1. Preterm Labor Risk (continued)

PARAMETER	FINDING	POINTS
Placenta previa during current pregnancy	Present	5
	Absent	0
Hydramnios during current pregnancy	Present	5
	Absent	0
Twins during current pregnancy	Present (probably multiple gestation)	5
	Absent	0
Abdominal surgery during current pregnancy	Present	10
	Absent	0

TOTAL SCORE	RISK OF PRETERM DELIVERY
0–5	Low risk
6–9	Intermediate risk
≥ 10	High risk

Total score is the sum total of points across all parameters:
Higher score = higher risk of preterm delivery.
Maximum possible is 50.

Tocolytics have not been proven to prolong pregnancy.

Tocolytic Agents
- IV magnesium sulfate—suppresses uterine contractions.
- Oral calcium channel blocker (nifedipine).
- β agonists (ritodrine, terbutaline)—stimulate β_2 receptors on myometrial cells → increased cyclic adenosine monophosphate (cAMP) → decreased intracellular Ca → decreased contractions.
  Side effects: Pulmonary edema, tachycardia, headaches.
- Prostaglandin inhibitors (indomethacin).
  Side effects: Premature constriction of ductus arteriosus, pulmonary HTN, and interventricular hemorrhage.

Mnemonic for contraindications to tocolysis: **BAD CHU**
- Severe **B**leeding from any cause
- Severe **A**bruptio placentae
- Fetal **D**eath/life-incompatible anomaly
- **C**horioamnionitis
- Severe pregnancy-induced **H**ypertension
- **U**nstable maternal hemodynamics

Contraindications to Tocolysis
- Severe **B**leeding from any cause
- Severe **A**bruptio placentae
- Fetal **D**eath/life-incompatible anomaly
- **C**horioamnionitis
- Severe pregnancy-induced **H**ypertension
- **U**nstable maternal hemodynamics

Magnesium Sulfate
- Unknown mechanism of action: Competes with calcium, inhibits myosin light chain.
- Side effects: Depressed reflexes, pulmonary edema, fatigue. Toxicity is treated with calcium gluconate.

Level	Side Effect
4–7 mg	Uterine contractions decreased
8–12 mg	Depressed deep tendon reflexes
> 12 mg	Respiratory/cardiac depression

Corticosteroids
- Given to patients in preterm labor from 24 to 34 weeks unless they have chorioamnionitis.
- Actions: Accelerate fetal lung maturity (decreases respiratory distress syndrome [RDS]), reduce intraventricular hemorrhage, and reduce necrotizing enterocolitis.

Assessing Fetal Lung Maturity
An amniocentesis may be performed to assess fetal lungs for risk of RDS. Fetal lungs are mature if:
- Phosphatidylglycerol is present in amniotic fluid

  or
- Lecithin–sphingomyelin ratio is > 2

PREMATURE RUPTURE OF MEMBRANES

Premature rupture denotes spontaneous rupture of fetal membranes *before the onset of labor.* This can occur at term (PROM) or preterm (PPROM).

- **ROM:** Rupture of membranes.
- **PROM:** Premature rupture of membranes (ROM before the onset of labor).
- **PPROM:** Preterm (< 37 weeks) premature rupture of membranes.
- **Prolonged rupture of membranes:** Rupture of membranes that lasts > 18 hours.

PROM is the most common diagnosis associated with preterm delivery.

Etiology

Unknown but hypothesized: Vaginal and cervical infections, incompetent cervix, abnormal membranes, nutritional deficiencies.

Risks

- *Prematurity:* If PROM occurs at < 37 weeks, the fetus is at risk of being born prematurely.
- *Oligohydramnios:* If PROM occurs at < 24 weeks, there is a risk of oligohydramnios (depleted amniotic fluid), which may cause **pulmonary hypoplasia.** *Survival at this age is low.*
- *Prolonged rupture of membranes:* The rupture of membranes > 18–24 hours before labor. Patients who do not go into labor immediately will have prolonged rupture of membranes and are at increasing risk of infection as the duration of rupture increases:
  - **Chorioamnionitis** and other infections.
  - Neonatal infection.
  - Umbilical cord prolapse.

Prolonged rupture of membranes can be caused by premature rupture (PROM) *or* an abnormally long labor (not PROM).

DIAGNOSIS OF PROM

The patient's history alone is correct in 90% of patients. Urinary leakage or excess vaginal discharge can be mistaken for PROM.

Nitrazine test may be falsely positive if contaminated with blood, semen, or vaginitis.

Diagnosis of Rupture of Membranes (ROM)

A digital exam should NOT be performed, as it increases the risk of infection:

- **Sterile speculum examination:**
  - Visualize extent of cervical effacement and dilation, and exclude prolapsed cord or protruding fetal extremity.
  - **Pool test:** Identify fluid coming from the cervix or pooled in the posterior fornix of the vagina → supports diagnosis of PROM.
- **Nitrazine test:** Put fluid on nitrazine paper, which turns blue if fluid is alkaline. Alkaline pH indicates fluid is amniotic.
- **Ferning test:** A swab from the posterior fornix is smeared on a slide, allowed to dry, and examined under a microscope for "ferning" (see Figure 9-2). This pattern is characteristic of amniotic fluid.

Management of All PROM Patients

- Evaluate patient for chorioamnionitis (common etiology of PROM): Fever > 38°C, leukocytosis, maternal/fetal tachycardia, uterine tenderness, malodorous vaginal discharge.
- If positive for chorioamnionitis, delivery is performed despite GA, and antibiotics are initiated (ampicillin, gentamicin).

Specific Management for PROM at Term

Ninety percent of term patients go into spontaneous labor within 24 hours after rupture:

- Patients in active labor should be allowed to progress.
- If labor is not spontaneous, it should be induced or cesarean delivery should be performed.

Specific Management of PPROM

Fifty percent of preterm patients go into labor within 24 hours after rupture.

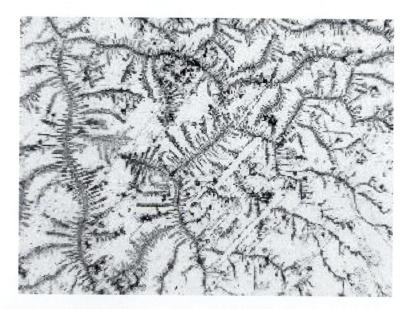

FIGURE 9-2. Ferning pattern.

Generally, one needs to balance the risks of premature birth against the risk of infection (which increases with the time that membranes are ruptured before birth).

- Amniotic fluid assessment of lecithin–sphingomyelin ratio for fetal lung maturity.
- Ultrasound to assess gestational age, position of baby, and amniotic fluid index.
- If < 34 weeks' gestation, give steroids to decrease incidence of respiratory distress syndrome.
- Antibiotic coverage to prolong latency.

THIRD-TRIMESTER BLEEDING

Incidence

Occurs in 2–5% of pregnancies.

Workup

- History and physical.
- Vitals.
- Labs: Complete blood count (CBC), coagulation profile, type and crossmatch, urinalysis, drug screen.
- Ultrasound.

See Figure 9-3 for management algorithm.

Determine whether blood is maternal or fetal or both:

- **Apt test:** Put blood from vagina in tube with KOH:
  - Turns brown for maternal.
  - Turns pink for fetus.
- **Kleihauer–Bettke test:** Take blood from mother's arm and determine percentage of fetal RBCs in maternal circulation: > 1% = fetal bleeding.
- **Wright's stain:** Vaginal blood; nucleated RBCs indicate fetal bleed.

Differential

Obstetric Causes
- Placental abruption
- Placenta previa
- Vasa previa/velamentous insertion
- Uterine rupture
- Circumvillate placenta
- Extrusion of cervical mucus ("bloody show")

Nonobstetric Causes
- Cervicitis
- Polyp
- Neoplasm

Golden rule: *Never* initially do a pelvic exam in a third-trimester bleed.

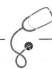

Apt, Kleihauer–Bettke, and Wright's stain tests determine if blood is fetal, maternal, or both.

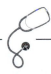

Placenta previa and abruption are the most common causes of third-trimester bleeding.

Complications of Pregnancy

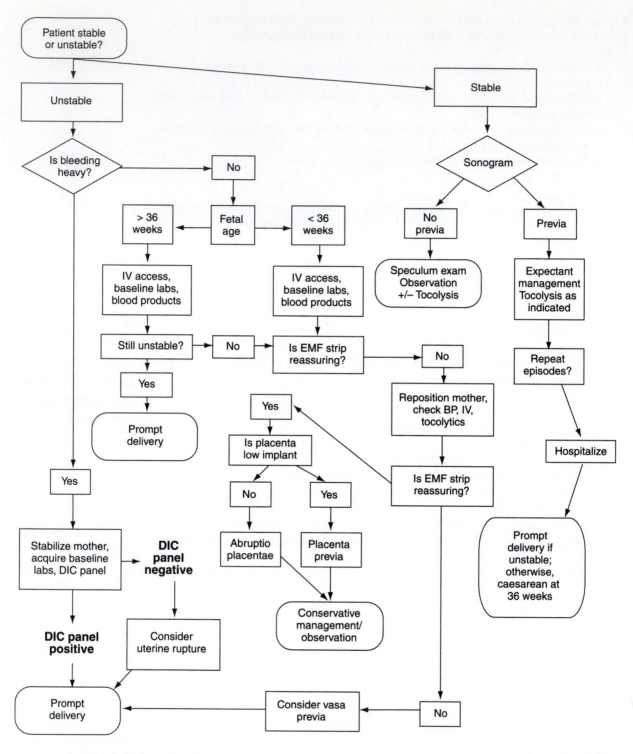

FIGURE 9-3. Third-trimester bleeding.

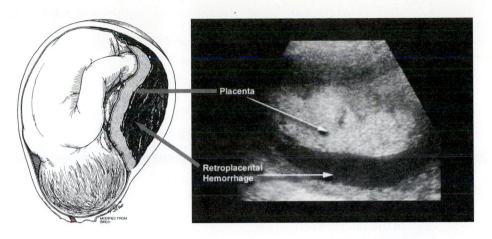

FIGURE 9-4. Placental abruption.

(Courtesy of SUNY at Buffalo School of Medicine, Residency Program in Emergency Medicine.)

Placental Abruption (Abruptio Placentae)

Premature separation of placenta from uterine wall before the delivery of baby (see Figure 9-4).

Incidence

0.5–1.3%; severe abruption leading to death (0.12%).

Risk Factors

- **Trauma** (usually shearing, such as a car accident).
- Previous history of abruption.
- **Preeclampsia (and maternal hypertension).**
- Smoking.
- Cocaine abuse.
- High parity.

Clinical Presentation

- Vaginal bleeding (maternal and fetal blood present).
- **Constant and severe back pain.**
- Irritable, tender, and typically hypertonic uterus.
- Evidence of fetal distress (if severe).
- Maternal shock.

Diagnosis

- Ultrasound will show retroplacental hematoma only part of the time.
- Clinical and pathological findings.

Management

- Correct shock (packed RBCs, fresh frozen plasma, cryoprecipitate, platelets).

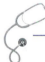

Most nonobstetric causes result in relatively little blood loss and minimal threat to the mother and fetus.

Pregnant woman + trauma + pain = abruption until proven otherwise.

Up to 20% of placental abruptions can present without vaginal bleeding because bleeding is internal.

- Expectant management: Close observation of mother and fetus with ability to intervene immediately.
- If there is fetal distress, perform C-section.

Placenta Previa (Figure 9-5)

A condition in which the placenta is implanted in the immediate vicinity of the cervical canal. It can be classified into four types:

- **Complete placenta previa:** The placenta covers the entire internal cervical os.
- **Partial placenta previa:** The placenta partially covers the internal cervical os.
- **Marginal placenta previa:** One edge of the placenta extends to the edge of the internal cervical os.
- **Low-lying placenta.**

Incidence

0.5–1%.

Etiology

Unknown, but associated with:

- Increased parity.
- Older mothers.
- Previous abortions.
- Previous history of placenta previa.
- Fetal anomalies.
- 5–10% associated with placenta accreta, especially if prior low transverse cesarean section.

Clinical Presentation

- **Painless,** profuse bleeding in T3.
- Postcoital bleeding.

Painless bleeding = Placenta Previa

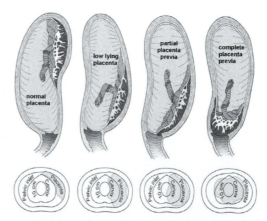

FIGURE 9-5.   A. Normal placenta. B. Low implantation. C. Partial placenta previa. D. Complete placenta previa.

(Reproduced, with permission, from DeCherney AH, Nathan L. *Current Obstetric & Gynecologic Diagnosis & Treatment,* 9th ed. New York: McGraw-Hill, 2003.)

HIGH-YIELD FACTS

Complications of Pregnancy

- Spotting during T1 and T2.
- Cramping (10% of cases).

Diagnosis

- **Transabdominal ultrasound** (95% accurate).
- **MRI findings:** Placenta previa is diagnosed on magnetic resonance imaging (MRI) when it is low lying and partially or completely covering the internal os. It is best demonstrated on sagittal images. The placenta appears homogeneous on MRI. On T1-weighted spin-echo images, it appears hypointense, with the intensity being marginally higher than that of the myometrium. T2-weighted spin-echo images demonstrate placental tissue as high signal intensity, which is distinct from the adjacent uterine tissue, fetus, and cervix.
- **Double set-up exam:** Take the patient to the operating room and prep for a C-section. Do speculum exam: If there is local bleeding, do a C-section; if not, palpate fornices to determine if placenta is covering the os. The double set-up exam is performed only on the rare occasion that the ultrasound is inconclusive and there is no MRI.

Management

Cesarean section is the delivery method of choice for placenta previa.

Fetal Vessel Rupture

Two conditions cause third-trimester bleeding resulting from fetal vessel rupture: (1) Vasa previa and (2) velamentous cord insertion. These two conditions often occur together.

Vasa Previa

A condition in which the fetal cord vessels unprotectedly pass over the internal os, making them susceptible to rupture and bleeding.

Incidence

0.03– 0.05%.

Presentation

Rapid vaginal bleeding and fetal distress (sinusoidal variation of fetal heart rate).

Management

Correction of shock and immediate C-section.

Velamentous Cord Insertion

The velamentous insertion of the umbilical cord into the fetal membranes: In other words, the fetal vessels insert between amnion and chorion. This leaves them susceptible to ripping when the amniotic sac ruptures.

Epidemiology

- 1% of single pregnancies
- 10% of twins
- 50% of triplets

Vaginal bleeding + sinusoidal variation of fetal heart rate = fetal vessel rupture/abruption.

RISK FACTORS FOR FETAL VESSEL RUPTURE

- Age > 30 years
- Prostaglandin induction
- Short interdelivery interval (18–24 months)
- Uterine scars
- Trauma
- Obstetric maneuvers
- Grand multiparity

Clinical Presentation

Vaginal bleeding with fetal distress.

Management

Correction of shock and immediate C-section.

Uterine Rupture

The ripping of the uterine musculature through all of its layers, usually with part of the fetus protruding through the opening.

Risk Factors

Prior uterine scar is the most important risk factor:
- Vertical scar: 10% risk
- Transverse scar: 0.5% risk

Presentation and Diagnosis
- **Sudden cessation of uterine contractions with a "tearing" sensation.**
- **Recession of the fetal presenting part.**
- Increased suprapubic pain and tenderness with labor (may not be readily apparent if analgesia/narcotics are administered).
- Vaginal bleeding (or bloody urine).
- Sudden, severe fetal heart rate deceleration.
- Sudden disappearance of fetal heart tones.
- Maternal hypovolemia from concealed hemorrhage.

Management
- May require a cesarean hysterectomy.
- If subsequent childbearing is important to the patient, rupture repair is possible but risky.

Other Obstetric Causes of Third-Trimester Bleeding

Circumvallate placenta: The chorionic plate (on fetal side of the placenta) is smaller than the basal plate (located on the maternal side), causing amnion and chorion to fold back onto themselves. This forms a ridge around the placenta with a central depression on the fetal surface.

Extrusion of cervical mucus ("bloody show"): A consequence of effacement and dilation of the cervix, with tearing of the small veins leading to slight shedding of blood. Treatment is rarely necessary.

All pregnant patients with a previous cesarean section must be consented for an elective "trial of labor" (vaginal delivery) with knowledge of the risk of uterine rupture:
- < 1% if previous low transverse C-section × 1
- < 2% if previous low transverse C-section × 2

Note: Previous classical C-section is a contraindication to vaginal birth after C-section.

ABNORMALITIES OF THE THIRD STAGE OF LABOR

Immediate Postpartum Hemorrhage
- Excessive bleeding that makes patient symptomatic and/or results in signs of hypovolemia.
- Blood loss > 500 mL in vaginal delivery; > 1,000 for C-section following delivery (difficult to quantify).

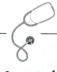

One unit of blood contains ≈ 500 mL.

- During first 24 hours: "Early" postpartum hemorrhage.
- Between 24 hours and 6 weeks after delivery: "Late" postpartum hemorrhage.

The most common cause is uterine atony. Normally, the uterus contracts, compressing blood vessels and preventing bleeding. Other causes of postpartum hemorrhage are summarized in the mnemonic CARPIT.

RISK FACTORS

- Blood transfusion/hemorrhage during a previous pregnancy
- Coagulopathy
- Vaginal birth after cesarean (VBAC)
- High parity
- Large infant/twins/polyhydramnios
- Midforceps delivery

MANAGEMENT

1. Manually compress and massage the uterus—controls most cases of hemorrhage due to atony.
2. Obtain assistance.
3. Give oxytocin (20 units in 1 L of lactated Ringer's) and methergonovine or prostaglandins if oxytocin is ineffective.
4. If not previously done, obtain blood for typing and crossmatching and begin volume resuscitation.
5. Carefully explore the uterine cavity to ensure that all placental parts have been delivered and that the uterus is intact.
6. Inspect the cervix and vagina for trauma/lacerations.
7. Place Foley and monitor urine output.

Causes of postpartum hemorrhage:

CARPIT
Coagulation defect
Atony of uterus
Rupture of uterus
Placenta retained
Implantation site bleeding
Trauma to genitourinary tract

If all this fails, consider:
- Hysterectomy
- Radiographic embolization of pelvic vessels
- Uterine artery ligation or hypogastric artery ligation

The cause of the postpartum bleeding should be sought out and treated immediately.

Abnormal Placentation

The abnormal implantation of the placenta in the uterus. These conditions can cause retention of the placenta after birth.

Types

- **Placenta accreta:** Placental villi attach directly to the myometrium rather than to the decidua basalis (see Figure 9-6).
- **Placenta increta:** Placental villi invade the myometrium.
- **Placenta percreta:** Placental villi penetrate through the myometrium.

Oxytocin should never be given as undiluted bolus because serious hypotension can result.

Etiology

These conditions are associated with:
- Placenta previa
- Previous C-section
- Previous dilation and curettage (D&C)
- Grand multiparity

Accreta = Attaches
Increta = Invades
Percreta = Penetrates

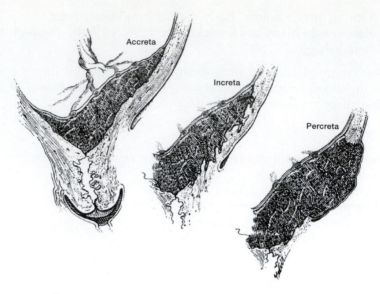

FIGURE 9-6. Placenta accreta, increta, and percreta.

(Reproduced, with permission, from Cunningham FG et al. *Williams Obstetrics*, 22nd ed. New York: McGraw-Hill, 2005: 831.)

Management

All of these conditions often result in postpartum hemorrhage (third stage of labor hemorrhage) and may require hysterectomy.

Uterine Inversion

This medical emergency most often results from an inexperienced person's pulling too hard when delivering the placenta. It can also be a result of abnormal placental implantation. Morbidity results from shock and sepsis.

Incidence

1/2,200 deliveries.

Management

- Administer anesthesia.
- Large-bore IV.
- Give blood PRN.
- Give uterine relaxants.
- Replace inverted uterus by pushing on the fundus toward the vagina.
- Oxytocin is given after uterus is restored to normal configuration and anesthesia is stopped.

Macrosomia

Defined as birth weight > 4,500 g:

Risk Factors

- Diabetes
- Obesity

- Previous history
- Post-term pregnancy
- Multiparity
- Advanced maternal age

Macrosomic infants are at risk for:
- Birth trauma
- Jaundice
- Hypoglycemia
- Low Apgar scores
- Childhood tumors

POSTPARTUM INFECTION

In the majority of instances, bacteria responsible for pelvic infections are those that normally reside in the bowel and colonize the perineum, vagina, and cervix.

Causes

Gram-positive cocci: Group A, B, and D streptococci
Gram-positive bacilli: *Clostridium* species, *Listeria monocytogenes*
Aerobic gram-negative bacilli: *Escherichia coli, Klebsiella, Proteus* species
Anaerobic gram-negative bacilli: *Bacteroides bovius, B. fragilis, B. disiens*
Other: *Mycoplasma hominis, Chlamydia trachomatis*

Risk Factors

- Prolonged rupture of membranes > 18 hours, prolonged second stage
- C-section/uterine manipulation
- Colonization of the lower genital tract with certain microorganisms (i.e., group B streptococci [GBS], *C. trachomatis*, *M. hominis*, and *Gardnerella vaginalis*)
- Premature labor
- Frequent vaginal exams
- Foreign body
- Diabetes

Diagnosis

- Fever > 100.4°F (38°C).
- Soft, tender uterus.
- Lochia has a foul odor.
- Leukocytosis (WBC > 10,000/µL) (remember physiologic leukocytosis; look for trends).
- Identify source of infection (urinalysis, culture of lochia).

Management

Broad-spectrum antibiotics.

The uterine cavity is sterile before rupture of the amniotic sac.

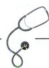

Endometritis is relatively uncommon following vaginal delivery, but 5–10 times more frequent after C-section.

Following delivery, the bladder and lower urinary tract remain somewhat hypotonic, resulting in residual urine and reflux, which predisposes to urinary tract infection.

GBS colonization leads to 80% greater likelihood of postpartum endometritis.

Types of Postpartum Infections

ENDOMETRITIS

Wound infection occurs in 4–12% of patients following C-section.

- A postpartum uterine infection involving the decidua, myometrium, and parametrial tissue.
- Also called *metritis with pelvic cellulitis, endomyometritis,* and *endoparametritis.*
- Typically develops postpartum day 2–3.
- Treat with IV antibiotics until patient is afebrile for 24–48 hours.
- GBS colonization increases risk of endometritis.

URINARY TRACT INFECTION

Antibiotic prophylaxis with IV cefazolin is commonly employed during C-section.

- Caused by catheterization, birth trauma, conduction anesthesia, and frequent pelvic examinations.
- Presents with dysuria, frequency, urgency, and low-grade fever.
- Rule out pyelonephritis (costovertebral angle tenderness, pyuria, hematuria).
- Obtain a urinalysis and urinary culture (*E. coli* is isolated in 75% of postpartum women).
- Treat with appropriate antibiotics.

CESAREAN SECTION WOUND INFECTION

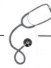

The more extensive the laceration/incision, the greater the chance of infection and wound breakdown.

- Fever and wound erythema and tenderness that persists to the fourth or fifth postoperative day suggests wound infection.
- Obtain Gram stain and cultures from wound material.
- Wound should be drained, irrigated, and debrided.
- Antibiotics should be given.

EPISIOTOMY INFECTION

- Look for pain at the episiotomy site, disruption of the wound, and a necrotic membrane over the wound.
- Rule out the presence of a rectovaginal fistula with a careful rectovaginal exam.
- Open, clean, and debride the wound to promote granulation tissue formation.
- Sitz baths are recommended.
- Reassess for possible closure after granulation tissue has appeared.

MASTITIS

Breast engorgement (painful, swollen, firm breasts) is *not* mastitis (due to infection) and is normal during the second to fourth postpartum day. Treat with supportive bra, 24-hour demand feedings, and ice packs if not breast-feeding.

Affects 1–2% of postpartum women. Two types: Epidemic (nosocomial) and nonepidemic:

- **Epidemic mastitis** is caused by infant acquiring *Staphylococcus aureus* in his nasopharynx from the hospital. Mother presents on day 2 to 4 with fever and breast tenderness. Treat with penicillin and isolate from other patients.
- **Endemic (nonepidemic) mastitis** presents weeks or months after delivery, usually during period of weaning. Mother presents with fever, systemic illness, and breast tenderness. Treat with penicillin or dicloxacillin. Continue breast-feeding.

Spontaneous Abortion, Ectopic Pregnancy, and Fetal Death

First-Trimester Bleeding	136
Spontaneous Abortion	136
Threatened Abortion	138
Inevitable Abortion	138
Incomplete Abortion	138
Complete Abortion	139
Missed Abortion	139
Septic Abortion	139
Recurrent Abortion	140
Ectopic Pregnancy	141
Fetal Death	144
Disseminated Intravascular Coagulation (DIC)	144

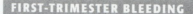

Differential Diagnosis

Approximately 30% of pregnancies result in spontaneous abortion.

- Spontaneous abortion.
- Ectopic pregnancy.
- Hydatidiform mole.
- Benign and malignant lesions (i.e., choriocarcinoma, cervical cancer).

Workup

- Vital signs (rule out shock/sepsis/illness).
- Pelvic exam (look at cervix, source of bleed).
- β-human chorionic gonadotropin (hCG) level, complete blood count (CBC).
- Ultrasound (US) (assess fetal viability; *abdominal US detects fetal heart motion by* ≥ *7 weeks' gestational age* [GA]).

Loss of a fetus of < 20 weeks' GA or weighing < 500 g = an "abortus."

See Figure 10-1 for management algorithm.

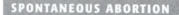

Spontaneous abortion is the termination of pregnancy resulting in expulsion of an immature, nonviable fetus:

- Occurs in 30% of all pregnancies.
- Most are unrecognized because they occur before or at the time of the next expected menses (70–80%).
- Fifteen to twenty percent of clinically diagnosed pregnancies are lost in T1 or early T2.

Sixty percent of spontaneous abortions in the first trimester are a result of chromosomal abnormalities.

Etiologies

Chromosomal Abnormalities

- Majority of abnormal karyotypes are numeric abnormalities as a result of errors during gametogenesis, fertilization, or the first division of the fertilized ovum.
- Frequency:
    - Trisomy: 50–60%
    - Monosomy (45,X): 7–15%
    - Triploidy: 15%
    - Tetraploidy: 10%

Infectious Agents

Infectious agents in cervix, uterine cavity, or seminal fluid can cause abortions. These infections may be asymptomatic:

Top etiologies of spontaneous abortion:
1. Chromosomal abnormalities
2. Unknown
3. Infection
4. Anatomic defects
5. Endocrine factors

- *Toxoplasma gondii*
- Herpes simplex
- *Ureaplasma urealyticum*
- *Mycoplasma hominis*
- *Listeria monocytogenes*
- Chlamydia
- Gonorrhea

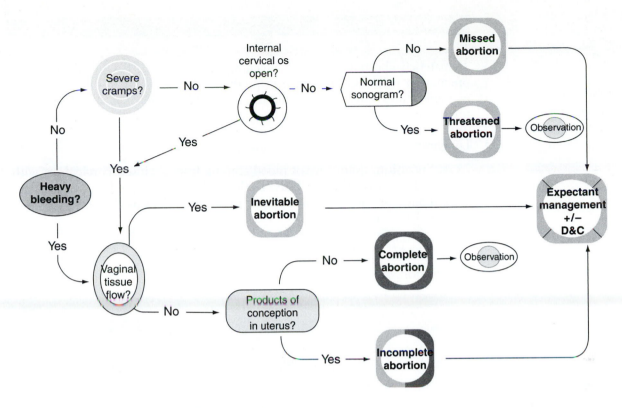

FIGURE 10-1. **Management of first-trimester bleeding.**

(Redrawn, with permission, from Lindarkis NM, Lott S. *Digging Up the Bones: Obstetrics and Gynecology.* New York: McGraw-Hill, 1998: 43.)

Uterine Abnormalities
- Septate/bicornuate uterus—25–30%
- Cervical incompetence
- Leiomyomas (especially submucosal)
- Intrauterine adhesions (i.e., from previous curettage)
- Trauma

Endocrine Abnormalities
- Progesterone deficiency
- Polycystic ovarian syndrome (PCOS)—hypersecretion of luteinizing hormone (LH)
- Diabetes—uncontrolled

Immunologic Factors
- Lupus anticoagulant
- Anticardiolipin antibody (antiphospholipid syndrome)

Environmental Factors
- Tobacco: ≥ 14 cigarettes/day increases abortion rates
- Alcohol
- Irradiation
- Environmental toxin exposure
- Caffeine: > 5 cups/day

Twenty to fifty percent of threatened abortions lead to loss of pregnancy.

THREATENED ABORTION

Threatened abortion is vaginal bleeding that occurs in the first 20 weeks of pregnancy, without the passage of products of conception (POC) or rupture of membranes. Pregnancy continues, although up to 50% result in loss of pregnancy.

Diagnosis

- Speculum exam reveals blood coming from a **closed cervical os, without amniotic fluid or POC in the endocervical canal.**
- Follow serial hCGs; should decrease by 65% every 48 hours (peaks at ~ 10 weeks).

Management

Observation.

INEVITABLE ABORTION

Inevitable abortion is vaginal bleeding, cramps, and **cervical dilation.** Expulsion of the products of conception (POC) is imminent.

Diagnosis

Speculum exam reveals blood coming from an **open** cervical os. Menstrual-like cramps typically occur.

Management

- Surgical evacuation of the uterus or expectant management (< 13 weeks).
- Rh typing—D immunoglobulin (RhoGAM) is administered to Rh-negative, unsensitized patients to prevent isoimmunization.

INCOMPLETE ABORTION

Incomplete abortion is the passage of some, but not all, POC from the cervical os.

Diagnosis

- Cramping and bleeding.
- Enlarged, boggy uterus.
- Dilated internal os with **POC present in the endocervical canal or vagina.**

Management

- Stabilization (i.e., IV fluids and oxytocin if heavy bleeding is present).
- Blood typing and crossmatching for possible transfusion if bleeding is brisk or low hemoglobin/patient symptomatic.

- RhoGAM if needed.
- POC are removed from the endocervical canal and uterus with ring forceps. Suction dilation and curettage (D&C) is performed after vital signs have stabilized.
- Karyotyping of POC if loss is recurrent.

COMPLETE ABORTION

Complete abortion is the complete passage of POC.

DIAGNOSIS

- Uterus is well contracted.
- Cervical os may be closed.
- Pain has ceased.

MANAGEMENT

- Examine all POC for completeness and characteristics.
- Between 8 and 14 weeks, curettage is often performed due to increased likelihood that the abortion was incomplete.
- Observe patient for further bleeding and fever.

MISSED ABORTION

Missed abortion is when the POC are retained after the fetus has expired.

Diagnosis

- The pregnant uterus fails to grow, and symptoms of pregnancy have disappeared.
- Intermittent vaginal bleeding/spotting/brown discharge and a firm, closed cervix.
- Decline in quantitative β-hCG.
- US confirms lack of fetal heartbeat.

Management

Although most women will spontaneously deliver a dead fetus within 2 weeks, the psychological stress imposed by carrying a dead fetus and the dangers of coagulation defects favor the practice of labor induction and early delivery:
- Check fibrinogen level, partial thromboplastin time (PTT), antibody screen, and ABO blood type.
- Evacuate the uterus (suction D&C in first trimester) or induce labor with IV oxytocin and cervical dilators or prostaglandin E_2 suppositories.
- Administer RhoGAM to Rh-negative, unsensitized patients.

SEPTIC ABORTION

- Infected products of conception (POC) are present.
- The infection is usually polymicrobial, often with *Staphylococcus aureus*, *Escherichia coli*, and other gram-negative organisms.

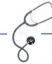

If POC are retained in septic abortion, severe sepsis often occurs.

Diagnosis

- Generalized pelvic discomfort, pain, and tenderness
- Signs of peritonitis
- Fever
- Malodorous vaginal and cervical discharge
- Leukocytosis

Management

- Cultures of uterine discharge and blood.
- Check CBC, urinalysis (UA), serum electrolytes, liver function tests (LFTs), blood urea nitrogen (BUN), creatinine, and coagulation panel.
- Abdominal and chest films to exclude free air in the peritoneal cavity (also helpful to look for the presence of gas-forming bacteria or foreign body).
- Prompt uterine evacuation (D&C), broad-spectrum IV antibiotics, IV fluids.

Consumptive coagulopathy is an uncommon but serious complication of septic abortion.

RECURRENT ABORTION

Three or more successive clinically recognized pregnancy losses prior to 20 weeks' GA constitutes recurrent abortion.

Women with two successive spontaneous abortions have a recurrence risk of 25–30%.

Etiology

- Parental chromosomal abnormalities (balanced translocation is the most common)
- Anatomic abnormalities (congenital and acquired)
- Endocrinologic abnormalities
- Infections (e.g., *Chlamydia, Ureaplasma*)
- Autoimmunity
- Unexplained (majority of cases)
- Maternal state hypercoagulable

Management

Investigate possible etiologies. Potentially useful tests include:

- Parental peripheral blood karyotypes
- Sonohysterogram (intrauterine structural study)
- Luteal-phase endometrial biopsy
- Anticardiolipin and antiphosphatidyl serine antibodies
- Lupus anticoagulant
- Factor V Leiden

See Table 10-1.

Recurrent abortion is three or more successive abortions.

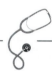

Women with a history of recurrent abortion have a 23% chance of abortion in subsequent pregnancies that are detectable by ultrasound.

A clinical investigation of pregnancy loss should be initiated after 2–3 successive spontaneous abortions in the first trimester or one in the second trimester.

TABLE 10-1. Types of Abortions

Complete abortion	Complete expulsion of POC before 20 weeks' gestation; cervix dilated.
Incomplete abortion	Partial expulsion of some POC before 20 weeks' gestation; partially dilated cervix.
Threatened abortion	No cervical dilatation or expulsion of POC; intrauterine bleeding before 20 weeks' gestation occurs.
Inevitable abortion	Threatened abortion with a dilated cervical os.
Missed abortion	Retention of nonviable POC for 4–8 weeks or more; often proceeds to complete abortion.
Recurrent spontaneous abortion	Three or more consecutive spontaneous abortions.
Septic abortion	Abortion associated with sepsis, severe hemorrhage, bacterial shock, and/or acute renal failure.
Therapeutic abortion (induced)	Termination of pregnancy before the period of fetal viability in order to protect the life or health of the mother.
Elective abortion (induced)	Termination of pregnancy before fetal viability at the request of the patient; not due to maternal or fetal health risks

ECTOPIC PREGNANCY

Ectopic pregnancy is the occurrence of conception outside of its normal position within the uterine cavity, the most common site being within the fallopian tubes (97%) followed by the abdominal cavity, ovary, and cervix. Within the fallopian tubes, the ampulla is the most common site, followed by the isthmus and fimbria (see Figure 10-2).

Ectopic pregnancy is the leading cause of pregnancy-related death during T1. Diagnose and treat *before* tubal rupture occurs to decrease the risk of death!

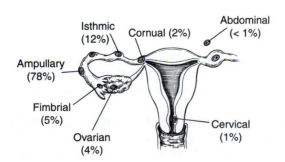

FIGURE 10-2. Sites of ectopic pregnancy.

(Reproduced, with permission, from Pearlman MD, Tintinalli JE, eds. *Emergency Care of the Woman.* New York: McGraw-Hill, 1998: 22.)

Epidemiology

- Rate of occurrence is 2% of reported pregnancies.
- Carries a 7- to 13-fold increase in recurrence risk.
- Three to four times more common in women over age 35 compared to those in the 15- to 24-year-old age group.

Etiology/Risk Factors

- Pelvic inflammatory disease (ask about history of sexually transmitted diseases [STDs]).
- Previous ectopic pregnancy.
- Previous tubal scarring (from surgery or tuberculosis).
- Salpingitis.
- Previous intrauterine device (IUD) use.
- Anatomic congenital malformations of the uterus such as septate uterus.
- Current smoking.
- Assisted reproduction measures such as use of ovulation-inducing drugs and in vitro fertilization.
- In utero diethylstilbestrol (DES) exposure.

Clinical Examination

- Pelvic exam may reveal normal or slightly enlarged uterus.
- Vaginal bleeding.
- Pelvic pain with manipulation of cervix.
- Palpable adnexal mass.
- Hemodynamic instability with generalized or rebound abdominal tenderness and guarding suggest rupture.

Diagnostic Tests

- Urine pregnancy test to confirm pregnancy: Will be positive with β-hCG levels > 20 mIU/mL, approximately 1 week after conception.
- β-hCG levels:
  - Should increase by at least 66% every 48 hours in the first 6–7 weeks of gestation after day 9.
  - Value of serial hCGs: Stable reliable patients can be followed with serial β-hCG levels. Inadequate rise in β-hCG is suggestive of ectopic or nonviable pregnancy.
- Progesterone (results often not available immediately):
  - > 25 ng/mL: Suggests normal intrauterine pregnancy (IUP).
  - < 5 ng/mL: Suggests abnormal pregnancy (either ectopic or nonviable pregnancy).
  - 5–25 ng/mL: unclear.
- Ultrasonography—diagnostic modality of choice:
  - Ectopic pregnancy is suspected if there is lack of visualization of the gestational sac within the uterine cavity in the setting of a positive pregnancy test.
  - Transvaginal sonography (TVUS) is more sensitive than transabdominal approach. The threshold for detecting an IUP on TVUS is β-hCG = 1,000 mIU/mL, or 4–6 weeks' gestation (see Figure 10-3).
  - Findings suggestive of ectopic pregnancy in addition to lack of the intrauterine gestational ring include ectopic gestational sac or cardiac activity, fluid or mass within the pouch of Douglas, and adnexal mass.

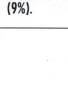

Ectopic pregnancy is the leading cause of pregnancy-related death (9%).

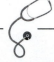

CLASSIC TRIAD OF ECTOPIC PREGNANCY
- Amenorrhea
- Vaginal bleeding
- Abdominal pain

Always do a pregnancy test in a woman of childbearing age with abdominal pain.

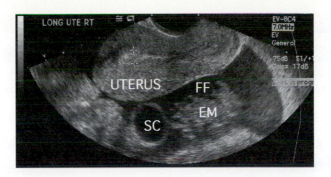

FIGURE 10-3. Transvaginal sonogram demonstrating an ectopic pregnancy.

Note the large amount of free fluid (FF) in the pelvis. No intrauterine pregnancy was seen. A large complex echogenic mass (EM) was seen in the left adnexa, consistent with an ectopic pregnancy. A simple cyst (SC) is also seen, in the right adnexa. The area within the uterus represents a small fibroid.

Differential

- Abortion
- Ovarian torsion
- Pelvic inflammatory disease (PID)
- Acute appendicitis
- Ruptured ovarian cyst
- Tubo-ovarian abscess

Management Options

General

- Resuscitative measures for all but the most stable patients, including two large-bore IVs, normal saline hydration, type and crossmatch.
- RhoGAM for all Rh-negative women.

Medical

Candidates for medical management with intramuscular methotrexate (folic acid antagonist) include:

- Asymtomatic women
- Serum β-hCG < 15,000 mIU/mL
- Ability for daily follow-up
- Tubal ring < 3 cm
- Absence of cardiac activity
- No hypersensitivity or medical contraindications to methotrexate therapy

Surgical

- Immediate intervention is warranted for symptomatic women with hemodynamic instability and patients who do not meet criteria for medical management.
- Laparoscopy with salpingostomy without fallopian tube removal is the preferred treatment.

β-hCG levels *do not* correlate with:
- Size of ectopic
- Potential for rupture
- Location of ectopic

Transvaginal IUP sonogram findings and corrresponding β-hCG thresholds:
- Gestational sac: ~ 1,000
- Yolk sac: ~ 2,500
- Heart tones: ~ 10,500

Do not coadminister a nonsteroidal anti-inflammatory drug (NSAID) with methotrexate, as it can potentiate nephrotoxicity.

FETAL DEATH

- Defined as death prior to complete expulsion or extraction from the mother, regardless of the duration of pregnancy.
- Can result in a spontaneous abortion and a missed abortion.

Causes

A carefully performed autopsy is the single most useful step in identifying the cause of fetal death.

T1 (1–14 Weeks)

The frequency of chromosomal abnormalities in stillbirths is 10 times higher than that in live births.

- **Chromosomal abnormalities**
- Environmental factors (e.g., medications, smoking, toxins)
- Infection (e.g., herpes simplex virus, human papillomavirus, mumps, *Mycoplasma*)
- Antiphospholipid antibodies (after 10 weeks)
- Maternal anatomic defects (e.g., maternal müllerian defects)
- Endocrine factors (e.g., progesterone insufficiency, thyroid dysfunction)
- Maternal systemic disease (e.g., diabetes)
- Unknown

T2 (14–28 Weeks)

- Anticardiolipin antibodies
- Antiphospholipid antibodies
- Chromosomal abnormalities
- Anatomic defects of uterus and cervix
- Infection (e.g., BV, syphilis)
- Erythroblastosis
- Placental pathological conditions (e.g., circumvallate placentation, placenta previa)

T3 (28 Weeks–Term)

Up to 35% of fetal deaths are associated with the presence of congenital malformation.

- Anticardiolipin antibodies
- Placental pathological conditions (e.g., circumvallate placentation, placenta previa, abruptio placentae)
- Infection

Time Nonspecific

- Trauma
- Cord entanglement
- Electric shock
- Maternal systemic disease
- Maternal infection

DISSEMINATED INTRAVASCULAR COAGULATION (DIC)

DIC or consumptive coagulopathy is a pathological condition associated with inappropriate activation of the coagulation and fibrinolytic system (i.e., thrombosis and hemorrhage). Most commonly, it is associated with one of the following disease states:

- Fetal demise
- Amniotic fluid embolism

- Preeclampsia–eclampsia
- Placental abruption
- Sepsis

Pathophysiology

In pathologic states (i.e., via thromboplastin production from dead POC), the coagulation cascade is activated, which results in consumption of platelets and coagulation factors. Fibrin deposition in small vessels results in bleeding and circulatory obstruction, which can lead to end-organ damage.

Diagnosis

- Physical exam may reveal multiple bleeding sites associated with purpura and petechiae.
- Lab evaluation reveals thrombocytopenia, hypofibrinogenemia, an elevated prothrombin time, increased fibrin split products, and hemolysis.

Management

Supportive therapy to correct/prevent shock, acidosis, and tissue ischemia; if applicable, prompt termination of pregnancy. Ultimately, the only care is to correct the underlying cause.

Pregnancy normally induces:
- Increases in coagulation factors I (fibrinogen), VII, VIII, IX, and X
- Increased activation of platelet clotting

In any obstetric complication, obtain a coagulation panel and fibrin split product levels to monitor for DIC.

Induced Abortion

Definition	148
Assessment of the Patient	148
Types of Induced Abortion	148
Indications for Therapeutic Abortion	148
Methods of Abortion	149
Less Common Methods of Abortion	149

The termination of a pregnancy medically or operatively before fetal viability; definition of viability varies from state to state.

ASSESSMENT OF THE PATIENT

Physical assessment is crucial before an elective abortion:
- **Ultrasound** should be performed if there is a discrepancy between dates and uterine size.
- Patient's **blood type and Rh type** must be evaluated; if Rh negative, RhoGAM should be administered prophylactically.
- Careful patient counseling should be performed.

TYPES OF INDUCED ABORTION

Elective voluntary: Interruption of pregnancy at the request of the mother.

Therapeutic: Interruption of pregnancy for the purpose of safeguarding the health of the mother.

INDICATIONS FOR THERAPEUTIC ABORTION

Maternal

- Cardiovascular disease
- Genetic syndrome (e.g., Marfan)
- Hematologic disease (e.g., thrombotic thrombocytopenic purpura [TTP])
- Metabolic (e.g., proliferative diabetic retinopathy)
- Neoplastic (e.g., cervical cancer; mother needs prompt chemotherapy)
- Neurologic (e.g., berry aneurysm; cerebrovascular malformation)
- Renal disease
- Intrauterine infection
- Severe preeclampsia/eclampsia

Fetal

- Major malformation (e.g., anencephaly)
- Genetic (e.g., spinal muscular atrophy)

First Trimester

MEDICAL

- Antiprogesterones such as mifepristone (RU 486), a prostaglandin analog, or epostane; used only before 9 weeks' gestation. Without progesterone, the uterine lining sloughs off.
- Methotrexate IM + vaginal misoprostol 1 week later; used only before 9 weeks' gestation. Methotrexate is a folic acid antagonist that interferes with cell division.

SURGICAL

Cervical dilation followed by aspiration curettage (D&C): Risks include cervical/uterine injury and Asherman syndrome, infection.

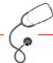

Mifepristone is useful only until 9 weeks because, after that, the placenta takes over production of progesterone.

Second Trimester

MEDICAL

Intravaginal prostaglandin E_2 (PGE_2) or $PGF_{2\alpha}$ with urea.

SURGICAL

Dilation and evacuation.

Complications of Surgical Abortions

- Infection
- Incomplete removal of products of conception (POC)
- Disseminated intravascular coagulation (DIC)
- Bleeding
- Cervical laceration
- Uterine perforation/rupture
- Psychological sequelae
- Death

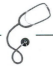

Medical methods of abortions can be used only in the first 49 days.

Medical

- Intra-amnionic infusion of hyperosmolar fluid (saline + urea).
- High-dose IV oxytocin (induces uterine contractions).

Surgical

- Hysterotomy is used only if other methods have been unsuccessful. A hysterotomy is a C-section of a preterm fetus.
- Hysterectomy.

What abortion method has the lowest complication rate? Dilation and evacuation. Risks include hemorrhage/perforation.

Death is a risk of abortion, but it is **10 times less** than the risk of death from giving birth.

HIGH-YIELD FACTS

Induced Abortion

NOTES

SECTION III

High-Yield Facts in Gynecology

► Contraception and Sterilization

► Infertility

► Menstruation

► Abnormal Uterine Bleeding

► Pelvic Pain

► Endometriosis and Adenomyosis

► Pelvic Masses

► Cervical Dysplasia

► Cervical Cancer

► Endometrial Cancer

► Ovarian Cancer

► Vulvar Dysplasia and Cancer

► Gestational Trophoblastic Neoplasia

► Sexually Transmitted Diseases and Vaginitis

► Vulvar Disorders

► Menopause

► Pelvic Relaxation

► Women's Health

Contraception and Sterilization

Contraception   154

Sterilization   159

General methods of preventing pregnancy include:

- Barrier
- Hormonal
- Intrauterine device (IUD)
- Sterilization
- Abstinence

Barrier Methods

FEMALE CONDOM

Rarely used because of expense and inconvenience (it must not be removed for 6–8 hours after intercourse). It offers labial protection, unlike the male condom. Efficacy 79%.

MALE CONDOM

Types
- Latex (cheapest and most common)
- Polyurethane (newest, sensitive, expensive)
- Animal skins (sensitive, least protection against sexually transmitted diseases [STDs])

Efficacy
86–97%, depending on if used properly.

Drawbacks
- Must be placed before contact
- Decreased sensation
- Rupture

The **only** contraceptive method that protects against STDs is the male condom.

DIAPHRAGM

A flexible ring with a rubber dome that must be fitted by a gynecologist: It forms a barrier from the cervix to the anterior vaginal wall. It must be inserted with spermicide and left in place after intercourse for 6–8 hours.

Types
- Flat or coil spring type (for women with good vaginal tone)
- Arching type (for poorer tone or vaginal/uteral irregularities such as cystoceles or long cervices)
- Wide seal rim

Efficacy
80–94%.

Complications
- If left in for too long, may result in *Staphylococcus aureus* infection (which may lead to **toxic shock syndrome**).
- May increase risk of urinary tract infection (UTI).

CERVICAL CAP

A smaller version of a diaphragm that fits directly over the cervix; more likely to cause irritation or toxic shock syndrome. It is more popular in Europe.

Efficacy
- In women who have not given birth: 80–90%
- In women who have given birth: 60–70%

SPERMICIDE

Foams, gels, creams placed in vagina up to 30 minutes before intercourse. Does not reduce the risk of STDs.

Types
Nonoxynol-9 and octoxynol-3; effective for only about 1 hour.

Efficacy
74–94%.

SPONGE

A polyurethane sponge containing nonoxynol-9 that is placed over the cervix: It can be inserted up to 24 hours before intercourse. Production has been discontinued in the United States.

Efficacy
84%.

Risk
Toxic shock syndrome.

Efficacy rates for spermicides are much higher when combined with other barriers (e.g., condoms, diaphragms).

Hormonal Agents

ORAL CONTRACEPTIVES (OCs)

Efficacy
95–99.9% (variability due to compliance).

Combination Pills

Contain estrogen and progestin; types include fixed dosing and phasic dosing:
- **Fixed dosing**: Requires the same dose every day of cycle.
- **Phasic dosing**: Gradual increase in amount of progestin as well as some changes in the level of estrogen.

Mechanism of Action
- **Estrogen** suppresses follicle-stimulating hormone (FSH) and therefore prevents follicular emergence.
- **Progesterone** suppresses the midcycle gonadotropin-releasing hormone (GnRH) surge, which suppresses luteinizing hormone (LH) and therefore prevents ovulation.
- Causes thicker cervical mucus.
- Causes decreased motility of fallopian tube.
- Causes endometrial atrophy.

Progestin-Only Pills

Contain only progestin: There is LH suppression and therefore no ovulation. The main differences from combination pills are:
- A mature follicle *is* formed (but not released).
- No placebo is used.

In combination oral contraceptives, at the time of desired/expected menstruation, a placebo is given to simulate the natural progesterone withdrawal.

Mechanism in a nutshell:
Estrogen inhibits FSH.
Progestin inhibits LH.

Estrogen suppresses breast milk, so combination pills are not used for nursing mothers. Progestin-only pills are used.

Oral contraceptives' link to an increase in breast cancer is not proven.

Why is estrogen a procoagulant? Estrogen increases factors VII and X and decreases antithrombin III.

Progestin-only pills are used in the following circumstances:

- Lactating women (progestin, unlike estrogen, does *not* suppress breast milk).
- Women > 40 years old.
- Women who cannot take estrogens for other medical reasons (e.g., estrogen-sensitive tumors).

Benefits of Oral Contraceptives

- Decreases risk of ovarian cancer by 75%.
- Decreases risk of endometrial cancer by 50%.
- Decreases bleeding and dysmenorrhea.
- Regulates menses.
- Reduces the risk of pelvic inflammatory disease (PID) (thicker mucus), fibrocystic breast change, ovarian cysts, ectopic pregnancy, osteoporosis, acne, and hirsutism.
- Decreases risk of anemia.

Risks of Oral Contraceptives

- Increased risk of venous thromboembolism/stroke (3/10,000).
- Increased risk of myocardial infarction (in smokers > 35 years old).
- Depression in some.
- Migraines.

Contraindications to Oral Combination Contraceptives

- Thromboembolism.
- History of ischemic stroke.
- Breast/endometrial cancer/estrogen dependent tumor.
- Cholestatic jaundice.
- Undiagnosed vaginal bleeding.
- Hepatic disease.
- Known/suspected pregnancy.
- Concomitant anticonvulsant therapy.
- Some antibiotics (efficacy of OCs is reduced by antibiotics, so an additional form of contraception should be used while taking them).
- Relative contraindications: Migraines, hypertension, lactation.
- Smokers > 35 years old.

Side Effects of Progestin-Only Oral Contraceptives

- Breakthrough bleeding
- Breast tenderness
- Nausea (10–30% of women)

INJECTABLE HORMONAL AGENTS

Medroxyprogesterone acetate (Depo-Provera) IM injection given every 3 months.

Efficacy
99.7%.

Mechanism of Action
Sustained high progesterone level to block LH surge (and hence ovulation). Thicker mucus and endometrial atrophy also contribute. There is no FSH suppression.

Indications
Especially suitable for women who either cannot tolerate OCs or who are unable to take OCs as prescribed, including:

- Seizures
- Mentally challenged

- Institutionalized
- Drug addiction

Side Effects of Injectable Hormonal Agents
- Bleeding irregularity/spotting
- Unknown when menstruation/fertility will resume after treatment cessation (can remain infertile for up to 6 months)
- Alopecia
- Mood changes
- Decreased high-density lipoprotein (HDL)
- Decreased libido

Contraindications
- Known/suspected pregnancy
- Undiagnosed vaginal bleeding
- Breast cancer
- Liver disease

IMPLANTABLE HORMONAL AGENTS

Subcutaneous implantation (inserted under the skin of the upper arm) of a rod containing levonorgestrel or etonorgestrel (a progesterol), which lasts about 3 years. No longer manufactured in the United States.

Efficacy
99.8%

Mechanism of Action
- Suppression of LH surge
- Thickened mucus
- Endometrial atrophy

Side Effects
- Irregular bleeding
- Acne
- Decreased libido
- Adnexal enlargement
- Possible difficult removal

Indications
- Oral contraceptives contraindicated/intolerated
- Smokers > 35 years old
- Women with diabetes mellitus, HTN, CAD

Contraindications
- Thrombophlebitis/embolism
- Known/suspected pregnancy
- Liver disease/cancer
- Breast cancer
- Concomitant anticonvulsant therapy

Intrauterine Device

Insertion of a T-shaped device (Paragard or Progestasert) into the endometrial cavity with a nylon filament extending through the cervix to facilitate removal.

Transdermal (Ortho Evra)
- Efficacy similar to combination OC.
- Better compliance.
- May come off and need replacement.

Vaginal ring (NuvaRing)
- Must be changed every 3 weeks.
- Must be inserted at the same time.
- Decreased efficacy if out > 3 hours.

Efficacy
97–99.1%.

Types
- Inert: Not used in the United States
- Paragard®: Made with copper; lasts 10 years
- Progestasert®: Releases progesterone; lasts 1 year
- Mirena®: Releases levonorgestrel; lasts 5 years

Mechanism of Action
- Copper prevents fertilization by creating a hostile environment (a sterile inflammatory reaction) for sperm and for a fertilized ovum.
- Prevents ovulation and causes endometrial atrophy (Progestasert® and Mirena®).
- Inhibit ovum fertilization and implantation.

Indications
- Oral contraceptives contraindicated/intolerated.
- Smokers > 35 years old.
- Mirena® can prevent menorrhagia.

Contraindications
- Multiple sexual partners
- History of PID
- Immunocompromised (e.g., HIV, sickle cell disease)
- Known/suspected pregnancy
- Wilson's disease
- Copper allergy

Complications
- PID
- Uterine perforation
- Ectopic pregnancy
- Menorrhagia and metrorrhagia (except levonorgestrel)
- IUD expulsion
- *Actinomyces*

The IUD filament provides access for bacteria, so there is a high risk for infection.

Copper and levonorgestrel reduce the risk of ectopic pregnancy compared to no contraceptives, but not as much as OCs.

Postcoital/Emergency Contraception

UP TO 3 DAYS AFTER INTERCOURSE

Levonorgestrel (Plan B): One 0.75-mg tablet taken within 72 hours of coitus. A second 0.75-mg tablet is taken 12 hours after the first dose. Efficacy: 89%.

UP TO 5 DAYS AFTER INTERCOURSE

Copper T IUD: Can be left in the uterine cavity and provide contraception for up to 10 years. Efficacy: Nearly 100%.

With about 1 million procedures per year in the United States, sterilization is the most popular form of birth control. There are 1–4 pregnancies per 1,000 sterilizations.

Male type: Vasectomy
Female type: Tubal obstruction

Tubal obstruction is twice as common as vasectomy.

Vasectomy

Excision of a small section of both vas deferens, followed by sealing of the proximal and distal cut ends. Ejaculation still occurs.

Sperm can still be found proximal to the surgical site, so to ensure sterility one must use contraception for 12 weeks or 20 ejaculations and then have two consecutive negative sperm counts.

Tubal Obstruction

Procedures can be performed either postpartum (immediately after delivery) or during an interval (between pregnancies).

LAPAROSCOPIC TUBAL OBSTRUCTION

Eighty to ninety percent of tubal obstructions are done laparoscopically. All methods occlude the fallopian tubes bilaterally.

Electrocautery

This involves the cauterization of a 3-cm zone of the isthmus. It is the most popular method (very effective but most difficult to reverse).

Clipping

The Hulka–Clemens clip (also Filshie clips), similar to a staple, is applied at a 90-degree angle on the isthmus. It is the most easily reversed method but also has the highest failure rate.

Banding

A length of isthmus is drawn up into the end of the trocar, and a silicone band, or Falope ring, is placed around the base of the drawn-up portion of fallopian tube.

HYSTEROSCOPIC OBSTRUCTION (ESSURE)

- New.
- Minimally invasive.
- Two-year data shows 99.8% efficacy.
- Alternative contraception needed until tubal occlusion proved by hysterosalpingogram.

Tubal obstruction facts:
- Electrocautery method is most popular and most difficult to reverse.
- Clipping method is most easily reversed but also the most likely to fail.

Pomeroy Method

A segment of isthmus is lifted and a suture is tied around the approximated base. The resulting loop is excised, leaving a gap between the proximal and distal ends. This is the most popular method.

Parkland Method

Similar to the Pomeroy but without the lifting, a segment of isthmus is tied proximally and distally and then excised.

Madlener Method

Similar to the Pomeroy but without the excision, a segment of isthmus is lifted and crushed and tied at the base.

Irving Method

The isthmus is cut, with the proximal end buried in the myometrium and the distal end buried in the mesosalpinx.

Kroener Method

Resection of the distal ampulla and fimbriae following ligation around the proximal ampulla.

Uchida Method

Epinephrine is injected beneath the serosa of the isthmus. The mesosalpinx is pulled back off the tube, and the proximal end of the tube is ligated and excised. The distal end is not excised. The mesosalpinx is reattached to the excised proximal stump, while the long distal end is left to "dangle" outside of the mesosalpinx.

PARTIAL OR TOTAL SALPINGECTOMY

Removal of part or all of the fallopian tube.

Luteal-Phase Pregnancy

A luteal-phase pregnancy is a *pregnancy diagnosed after tubal sterilization but conceived before*. Occurs around 2–3/1,000 sterilizations. It is prevented by either performing sensitive pregnancy tests prior to the procedure or performing the procedure during the follicular phase.

Reversibility of Tubal Obstruction

Around one third of tubal ligations can be reversed such that pregnancy can result. **Pregnancies after reversal are ectopic until proven otherwise, and therefore reversal does not preclude a full ectopic workup.**

Complications of Tubal Obstruction

- Failure of procedure (patient still fertile).
- **Poststerility syndrome:** Pelvic pain/dysmenorrhea, menorrhagia, ovarian cyst.
- **Fistula formation:** Uteroperitoneal fistulas can occur, especially if the procedure is performed on the fallopian tubes < 2–3 cm from the uterus.
- Infection.
- Operative complications.

Other Methods of Sterilization

COLPOTOMY

Utilizes entry through the vaginal wall near the posterior cul-de-sac and occludes the fallopian tubes by employing methods similar to those performed in laparoscopy and laparotomy.

HYSTERECTOMY

Removal of the uterus, either vaginally or abdominally; rarely performed for sterilization purposes. Failure rate is < 1%. **Pregnancy after hysterectomy = ectopic pregnancy = emergency.**

NOTES

Infertility

Definition	164
Female Factors Affecting Infertility	164
Infertility Workup	164
Assisted Reproductive Technologies	166

- Female factors account for 40–50% of infertile couples.
- Male factors account for 23% of infertile couples.
- In 40% of infertile couples, there are multiple causes.

Calcium channel blockers and furantoins can impair sperm function and quantity.

DEFINITION

- The inability to conceive **after 12 months** of unprotected sexual intercourse.
- Affects 15% of couples.

Types

Primary infertility: Infertility in the absence of previous pregnancy.
Secondary infertility: Infertility after previous pregnancy.

FEMALE FACTORS AFFECTING INFERTILITY

- Tubal disease: 14%
- Anovulation: 18%
- Unexplained: 28%
- Endometriosis: 9%
- Multifactorial: 40%

INFERTILITY WORKUP

See Table 13-1.

Semen Analysis

Performed after at least 48 hours of abstinence, with examination maximum 2 hours from time of ejaculation (for those who prefer to collect at home).

CHARACTERISTICS

- Volume: Normal, > 2 mL
- Semen count: Normal, ≥ 20 million/mL
- Motility: Normal, > 50% with forward movement
- Morphology: Normal, > 40%

TABLE 13-1. Evaluation of Infertile Couple

Male factor: Semen analysis.
Ovulation factor: Serum progesterone, endometrial biopsy.
Cervical factor: Postcoital test.
Uterine factor: Ultrasonography, hysterosonogram, hysterosalpingogram, hysteroscopy.
Tubal factor: Hysterosalpingogram, laparoscopy.
Endometriosis: Laparascopy.

TREATMENT FOR ABNORMAL SPERM FINDINGS

- Depends on the cause
- Urology referral
- Quitting smoking, EtOH
- Avoidance of lubricants
- Clomiphene 25 mg/day for 25 days, with 5 days of rest
- Intrauterine insemination (sperm injected through cervix)
- Intracytoplasmic sperm injection
- Artificial insemination

If semen analysis is normal, continue workup with assessment of ovulation.

Methods of Assessing Ovulation

- **History of monthly menses** is a strong indicator of normal ovulation.
- **Basal body temperature (BBT)**: Body temperature rises about 0.5–1°F during the luteal phase due to the increased level of progesterone. Presence of BBT increase is a good indicator that ovulation is occurring. (See Figure 14-1, page 171.)
- Measurement of **luteal-phase progesterone** level (normal, 4 ng/mL) and luteinizing hormone/follicle-stimulating hormone (LH/FSH) ratio for polycystic ovarian syndrome (PCOS).
- **Salpingogram/sonogram**: Determines normal or abnormal endometrial and tubal anatomy and PCOS.
- **Endometrial biopsy**: Determines histologically the presence/absence of ovulation.

POSSIBLE CAUSES AND TREATMENTS OF ANOVULATION

- **Pituitary insufficiency:** Treat with intramuscular (LH/FSH) or clomiphene.
- **Hypothalamic dysfunction:** Treat with bromocriptine (a dopamine agonist).
- **PCOS:** Treat with clomiphene +/– metformin.
- **Other causes:** Hyper/hypothyroid, androgen excess, obesity/starvation, galactorrhea, stress.

If ovulation analysis and semen analysis are normal, analysis of the internal architecture is performed to determine if there is an anatomical impediment to pregnancy. In most cases, an internal architecture study is part of the initial workup.

Internal Architecture Study

HYSTEROSALPINGOGRAM

- Performed during follicular phase.
- Radiopaque dye is injected into the cervix and uterus and should fill both fallopian tubes and spill into the peritoneal cavity.
- Allows visualization of uterus and fallopian tubes.
- There is a risk of salpingitis from the injection.

- Basal body temperature (BBT) must be taken first thing in the morning. A monthly rise in BBT indicates ovulation is occurring.
- Ovulation = highest temperature of month.

Clomiphene: An antiestrogen that inhibits negative feedback on the central nervous system or induces ovulation by simulating the release of pituitary gonadotropins.

Hysterosalpingogram is neither sensitive nor specific (smooth muscle spasm occludes tubes) for determining the presence of anatomical problems.

Endometriosis and unexplained infertility account for 25% of infertile couples. Endometriosis may be present in 40% of these couples.

TREATMENT FOR STRUCTURAL ABNORMALITIES

- Microsurgical tuboplasty
- Neosalpingostomy
- Tubal reimplantation for intramural obstruction
- In vitro

If findings of the semen analysis, ovulation analysis, and hysterosalpingogram are normal, an exploratory laparoscopy can be done.

Exploratory Laparoscopy

A laparoscope is inserted transabdominally to visualize the pelvis:
- Check for adhesions.
- Check for endometriosis.
- Check for tubal anomalies.

TREATMENT

- Laparoscopic lysis of adhesions
- Laparoscopic endometriosis ablation
- Medical treatment of endometriosis

ASSISTED REPRODUCTIVE TECHNOLOGIES

Definition

Directly retrieving eggs from ovary followed by manipulation and replacement: **Generally employed for inadequate spermatogenesis.** The following are examples.

Intracytoplasmic Sperm Injection (ICSI)

ICSI is reserved for moderate to severe male infertility.

- Revolutionized treatment of infertility in men with severe oligospermia, azoospermia, asthenospermia (low motility), teratospermia (abnormal morphology).
- Injection of spermatozoon into oocyte cytoplasm.
- Pregnancy rate: 20% per cycle.
- Multiple pregnancy rate: 28–38%.
- Not influenced by cause of abnormal sperm.
- Can use spermatozoa from testicular biopsies.
- Expensive.

In Vitro Fertilization (IVF) and Embryo Transfer

Fertilization of eggs in a lab followed by uterine placement: ICSI is a subtype of IVF to aid severe male factors. Success rate of IVF is about 20%.

Artificial Insemination of Donor Sperm

Success rate is 75% in six cycles.

Gamete Intrafallopian Transfer (GIFT)

Egg and sperm placement in an intact fallopian tube for fertilization: Success rate of GIFT is about 25%.

Zygote Intrafallopian Transfer (ZIFT)

Zygote (fertilized in vitro) is created and placed in fallopian tube, where it proceeds to uterus for natural implantation: Success rate of ZIFT is about 30%.

HIGH-YIELD FACTS

Infertility

Menstruation

Development   170

The Menstrual Cycle   170

Amenorrhea   172

Hyperprolactinemia   173

Premenstrual Syndrome (PMS)   174

Some Most Commons   175

Androgen Excess, Hirsutism, and Virilism   175

Average thelarche—10 years old due to ↑ estradiol

Average pubarche—11 years old due to ↑ adrenal hormones

Average menarche—12 years old due to ↑ estradiol

Puberty

Puberty is the transition from childhood to reproductive potential. More commonly, it refers to the final stage of maturation known as adolescence.

Puberty is believed to begin with *disinhibition* of the pulsatile gonadotropin-releasing hormone (GnRH) secretion from the hypothalamus (mechanism is unknown).

SECONDARY SEX CHARACTERISTICS

Development of the secondary sexual characteristics proceeds in the following order:

1. Breast budding (thelarche)
2. Axillary and pubic hair growth (pubarche)
3. First menses (menarche)

TANNER STAGES

Tanner stages:
Stage 1: Prepubertal child
Stages 2–4: Developmental stages
Stage 5: Adult

The Tanner stages of development refer to the sequence of events of breast and pubic hair development.

Precocious Puberty

Appearance of the secondary sexual characteristics before 8 years of age is referred to as precocious puberty and requires investigation into the etiology.

Etiology (Not an Exhaustive List)

- Idiopathic (most common).
- Tumors of the hypothalamic–pituitary stalk (prevent negative feedback).
- Inflammation of the hypothalamus (increased gonadotropin-releasing hormone [GnRH] production).
- 21-hydroxylase deficiency.
- Estrogen-secreting tumors.
- Excess exogenous estrogen.

Many follicles are stimulated by FSH, but *the follicle that secretes more estrogen than androgen will be released.* This dominant follicle releases more and more estradiol so that its positive feedback causes an LH surge.

The menstrual cycle is the cyclical changes that occur in the female reproductive system (see Figure 14-1): The hypothalamus, pituitary, ovaries, and uterus interact to cause ovulation approximately once per month (average 28 days [+/− 7 days]).

Days 1–4: First Part of the Follicular Phase

- In the absence of fertilization, **progesterone withdrawal results in endometrial sloughing** (menses).
- Prostaglandins contained in those endometrial cells are released, often resulting in cramps from uterine contractions.
- Ovaries quiescent.

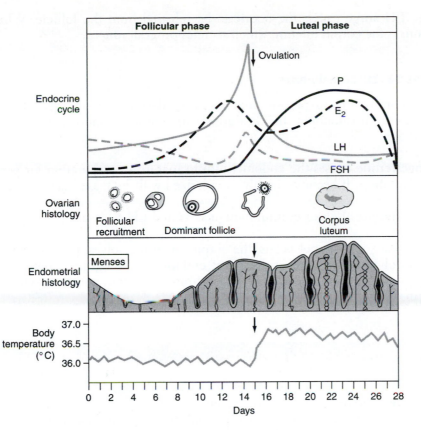

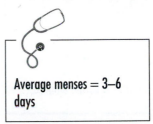

Average menses = 3–6 days

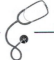

Blood loss in menstruation averages 30–50 mL, should not form clots. > 80 mL is an abnormal amount of blood loss.

FIGURE 14-1. The menstrual cycle.

(Modified, with permission, from Fauci AS, Braunwald E, Isselbacher KJ, et al. *Harrison's Principles of Internal Medicine*, 14th ed. New York: McGraw-Hill, 1998: 2101.)

Days 1–14: Follicular (Proliferative) Phase

The follicular phase begins on the first day of menses. Now that progesterone levels have fallen with the regression of the corpus luteum, all hormone levels are low. Without any negative feedback, **GnRH** from the hypothalamus causes follicle-stimulating hormone (**FSH**) levels to rise.

FSH released from the pituitary stimulates maturation of granulosa cells in the ovary. The granulosa cells secrete **estradiol** in response.

Estradiol inhibits luteinizing hormone (**LH**) and **FSH** due to negative feedback. In the meantime, the **estradiol** secretion also causes the endometrium to proliferate.

LH acts on the theca cells to increase secretion of **androgens** (which are converted to estradiol), prepare the cells for progesterone secretion, and cause further granulosa maturation.

Day 14: Ovulation

Estradiol peaks 1 day prior to ovulation. At this point, there is a unique phenomenon. The negative feedback on **LH** switches to a positive feedback, thus the **LH surge** (other factors also play a role).

Main event of menstruation: Absence of progesterone causes endometrial sloughing.
Two main events in follicular phase:
- FSH causes follicle maturation and estrogen secretion.
- Estrogen causes endometrial proliferation.

Main event of ovulation: LH surge causes oocyte to be released.

Main events of luteal phase: Corpus luteum secretes progesterone, which causes:
- Endometrial maturation
- ↓ FSH, ↓ LH

The **LH surge** causes the oocyte to be released from the follicle. What remains is the corpus luteum, which secretes **progesterone**.

Days 14–28: Luteal Phase

The corpus luteum persists only about 11 days in the absence of human chorionic gonadotropin (hCG), during which time it continues **progesterone** secretion.

Progesterone causes the endometrium to mature in preparation for possible implantation. It becomes highly vascularized with increased gland secretion.

Progesterone also causes inhibition of **FSH** and **LH** release.

If fertilization does not occur, the corpus luteum resolves, **progesterone** and **estradiol** levels fall, with subsequent endometrial sloughing (menses). The hypothalamic–pituitary axis is released from inhibition, and the cycle begins again.

The corpus luteum is maintained after fertilization by hCG, released by the embryo.

Absence of menses for 3–6 months is defined as **oligomenorrhea.**

When diagnosing amenorrhea, always rule out pregnancy first.

Uterine causes have normal levels of FSH/LH.

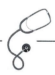

Progestin challenge test: Give progestin for 5 days and then stop. This stimulates progesterone withdrawal. If ovaries are secreting estrogen, sloughing will occur and menses results. No menses indicates no ovaries, no estrogen, or blood flow obstruction.

AMENORRHEA

- **Primary amenorrhea:** Absence of menses by age 16.
- **Secondary amenorrhea:** Absence of menses for ≥ 6 months in a woman who previously had normal menses. The most common cause is pregnancy.

Etiologies

Hypothalamic Causes

All hypothalamic causes result in decreased FSH/LH levels:
- **Kallmann syndrome:** Congenital lack of GnRH.
- **Pituitary stalk compression:** Tumors, granulomas, irradiation.
- **Decreased GnRH release:** Stress, anorexia, hyperprolactinemia, severe weight loss, extreme exercise.

Pituitary Causes

All pituitary causes result in decreased FSH/LH levels:
- **Sheehan syndrome:** Pituitary infarction resulting from hypotension during delivery, usually resulting from hemorrhage.
- **Tumors:** Either compress stalk (as above) or secrete prolactin.
- **Hemosiderosis:** Iron deposition in pituitary that impairs its function.
- Thyroid disease.

Ovarian Causes

All ovarian causes result in increased FSH/LH levels:
- **Premature ovarian failure:** Menopause before age 35, chemotherapy.
- **Savage syndrome:** Ovarian resistance to FSH/LH.
- **Enzyme defects:** Most commonly 17α-hydroxylase deficiency.
- **Turner syndrome** (XO karyotype): Ovarian dysgenesis.
- **Polycystic ovarian syndrome (PCOS):** Increased estrogen levels cause increased LH levels, resulting in abnormal follicular growth and androgen secretion.

Mechanical Causes

- Imperforate hymen
- Abnormal müllerian development
- **Asherman syndrome:** Uterine scarring and adhesions following dilation and curettage (D&C)
- Transverse vaginal septum
- Other causes:
  - Androgen insensitivity
  - Abnormal müllerian development

Evaluation

See Figure 14-2.

Treatment

Hypothalamic Causes

- Tumor removal
- Weight gain
- Stress relief
- Exogenous pulsatile GnRH

Pituitary Causes

- Tumor removal
- Bromocriptine (dopamine agonist inhibits prolactin release)
- Exogenous FSH/LH

Ovarian Causes

- Ovarian failure: Hormone replacement therapy
- PCOS: Clomiphene (an antiestrogen) +/– metformin

Mechanical Causes

- Obstruction: Surgery

GnRH is associated with an increased risk of osteoporosis. The current recommendation is to take it for only 6 months.

Early menopause is idiopathic.

PCOS patients are usually obese and have hirsutism and insulin resistance. It is the most common cause of hirsutism.

HYPERPROLACTINEMIA

Elevated prolactin levels could be due to:

- Hypothyroidism: Check TSH level (hypothyroidism causes a rise in prolactin).
- Central nervous system (CNS) tumors: Perform head computed tomography (CT)/magnetic resonance imaging (MRI).
- Drugs:
  - Dopamine antagonists (antipsychotics)
  - Methyldopa
  - Serotonin agonists
  - Verapamil
- Spinal cord lesions: Perform spinal CT/MRI.
- Nipple stimulation (breast-feeding).
- Decreased prolactin clearance.
- Idiopathic.

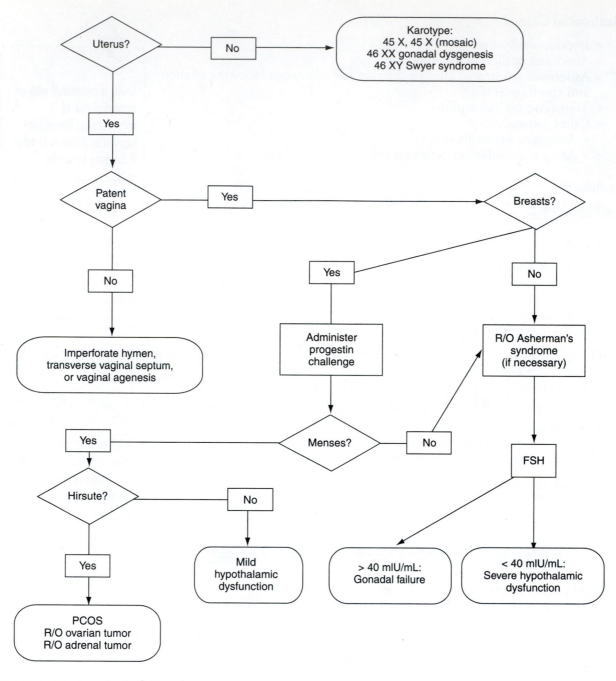

FIGURE 14-2. Amenorrhea workup.

PMS refers to a group of symptoms experienced during the luteal phase of the menstrual cycle. Affects up to 75% of women.

Symptoms may manifest as:
- **Somatic complaints:** Headaches, bloating, breast tenderness, fatigue.
- **Emotional changes:** Anxiety, depression, irritability.

- **Behavior symptoms:** Trouble concentrating, food cravings, sleep changes, mood lability, fatigue.

Premenstrual Dysphoric Disorder (PMDD)

- Most severe form of PMS
  - Anger
  - Irritability
  - Internal tension
- Affects 3–8% of women

Management of PMS

- Diet: Luteal-phase reductions in alcohol, caffeine, fats, tobacco, refined sugars: Decreases irritability by decreasing fluctuation in blood sugar levels.
- Sodium restriction: Decreases edema.
- Oral contraceptive pills: Cause anovulation, which improves symptoms.
- Nonsteroidal anti-inflammatory drugs (NSAIDs): Decrease inflammation found in PMS.
- Selective serotonin reuptake inhibitors (SSRIs).
- GnRH agonists.

SOME MOST COMMONS

- **Most common method of family planning:** Tubal sterilization.
- **Most common reason for neonatal sepsis:** Chorioamnionitis (group B *Streptococcus, Escherichia coli*).
- **Most common reason for hospitalization in women of reproductive age:** Endometriosis.
- **Most common postoperative complication:** Pulmonary atelectasis.
- **Most common cause of primary amenorrhea:** Gonadal dysgenesis.
- **Most common cause of fetal morbidity and mortality:** Preterm labor.

ANDROGEN EXCESS, HIRSUTISM, AND VIRILISM

Androgens

Androgens are steroid hormones produced in the gonads (ovaries in women, the testes in males) and in the adrenal glands.

EFFECTS OF ANDROGEN EXCESS: HIRSUTISM AND VIRILIZATION

Androgens promote hair growth at puberty, although to different extents in each sex. Females, with low levels of androgens, develop visible pubic and axillary hair. Males, with greater concentrations of androgen, get additional hair growth on the face and chest, as well as masculinization (i.e., increased muscle mass, broadening of shoulders, and deepening of the voice).

Excess androgen in women will also result in these changes as well. In this context, these effects are termed *hirsutism* and *virilism*.

Hirsutism—the development of increased terminal hairs on the chest, abdomen, and face in a woman.

Virilization—the development of masculine characteristics in a woman, such as deepening of the voice, clitoromegaly, loss of female body contour, decreased breast tissue, and male pattern balding.

Hair Types

Vellus hairs are fine hairs found on most parts of the body. They are barely visible. **Terminal hairs** are the coarse, darker hairs found, for example, in the axilla and pubic region. Androgens facilitate the conversion of vellus to terminal hairs.

PRODUCTION OF ANDROGENS

In women, androgens are produced in two locations: The adrenals and the ovaries (in males, they are produced in the adrenals and testes).

ADRENAL PRODUCTION OF ANDROGENS

The **zona fasciculata** and the **zona reticularis** of the adrenal cortex produce androgens, as well as cortisol. ACTH regulates production.

A third layer of the adrenal cortex, the **zona glomerulosa,** produces aldosterone and is regulated by the renin–angiotensin system.

All three hormones—cortisol, androgens, and aldosterone—are derived from cholesterol. Androgen products from the adrenal are found mostly in the form of dehydroepiandrosterone (DHEA) and dehydroepiandrosterone sulfate (DHEA-S). Elevation in these products represents increased adrenal androgen production.

OVARIAN PRODUCTION OF ANDROGENS

In the ovaries, first, LH stimulates the theca cells to produce androgens (androstenedione and testosterone). Then, FSH stimulates granulosa cells to convert these androgens to estrone and estradiol. When LH levels become disproportionately greater than FSH levels, androgens become elevated.

Pathologies

Excess androgen can be either ovarian etiology or adrenal, neoplastic, or benign.

Adrenal Etiologies

Cushing Syndrome and Cushing Disease
- **Cushing syndrome** is a general term meaning hypercortisolism along with the clinical picture that goes with it—moon face, buffalo hump, weakness, etc. Exogenous or endogenous cortisol can be the cause.
- **Cushing disease** is a subset of Cushing syndrome, in which the increased cortisol level is due to ACTH hypersecretion by the pituitary, usually secondary to a benign pituitary adenoma. It accounts for 70% of

CORTISOL PRODUCTION IN THE ADRENALS
Where? Zonas fasciculata and reticularis
Regulated by? ACTH
Derived from? Cholesterol

DHEA and DHEA-S are androgen products from the adrenals. Increased levels of these indicate that the source is adrenal.

High LH:FSH ratio in the context of androgen excess indicates that ovary is the source.

Cushing syndromes. Virilism and hirsutism are associated with this condition because the ACTH stimulates androgen production as well.

- **Paraneoplastic syndromes** in which tumors (usually small cell lung cancer) produce ectopic ACTH are another cause of increased cortisol. These account for 15% of Cushing syndromes.
- **Adrenal tumors** (adenoma or carcinoma) account for the remaining 15% of Cushing syndromes. In general, adenomas produce only cortisol, so no hirsutism or virilization is present. Carcinomas, by contrast, often produce androgens as well as cortisol, so they may present with signs of hirsutism and virilization.

Congenital Adrenal Hyperplasias

Congenital adrenal hyperplasia is a general term for disease entities involving defects in steroid, androgen, and mineral corticoid synthesis. Two such common entities that result in virilism and hirsutism due to increased androgens are 21-hydroxylase deficiency and 11β-hydroxylase deficiency.

- **21-Hydroxylase deficiency**: This is the most common congenital adrenal hyperplasia. The condition has various levels of severity. Affected individuals lack an enzyme crucial to cortisol and mineral corticoid production. Therefore, hormone synthesis is shunted to excessive production of androgens. Elevated serum 17-hydroxyprogesterone levels are found as well. In the severe form, affected females have ambiguous genitalia at birth, along with severe salt wasting and cortisol insufficiency. A milder form presents simply with virilization and hirsutism of females after puberty.
- **11β-Hydroxylase deficiency**: This condition is associated with decreased cortisol, but increased mineral corticoids and androgens. The resultant picture is a severe hypertension with virilization/hirsutism (which results in pseudohermaphroditism of female babies). 11-Deoxycortisol levels are high.

Ovarian Etiologies

Polycystic Ovarian Syndrome (PCOS)

PCOS is a common condition (affecting 5% of reproductive age women) and is characterized by hirsutism, virilization, amenorrhea, obesity, and diabetes (sometimes). Ovaries are found to have multiple inactive cysts with hyperplastic ovarian stroma. The LH:FSH ratio is often greater than 3:1. The cause is unknown, and the treatment is oral contraceptives +/− metformin.

Hyperthecosis

Hyperthecosis is when an area of luteinization occurs in the ovary, along with stromal hyperplasia. The luteinized cells produce androgens: Hirsutism and virilization may result.

Theca Lutein Cysts

As described above, theca cells produce androgens and granulosa cells transform the androgens to estrogens. Theca lutein cysts produce abnormally high levels of androgens, in excess of the amount that can be converted to estrogens. Diagnosis is made by ovarian biopsy.

21-Hydroxylase deficiency typical scenario:
A baby with ambiguous genitalia, dangerously hypotensive, and with elevated 17-hydroxyprogesterone.

11β-Hydroxylase deficiency:
Low cortisol, high mineral corticoids (hypertensive) and high androgens.
11-Deoxycortisol is elevated.
vs.
21-Hydroxylase deficiency:
Low cortisol and mineral corticoids (hypotensive), high androgens.
17-Hydroxyprogesterone is elevated.

A 24-year-old obese woman with facial hair comes in with complaints of amenorrhea. LH:FSH ratio is elevated. *Think:* PCOS.

A baby with ambiguous genitalia is born to a mother who complains of increased facial hair growth over last few months. *Think: Luteoma of pregnancy.*

Luteoma of Pregnancy

Luteoma of pregnancy is a benign tumor that grows in response to human chorionic gonadotropin. Virilization may occur in both the mother and the female fetus. The tumor usually disappears postpartum, as do the clinical features.

Androgen-Secreting Ovarian Neoplasms

Sertoli–Leydig cell tumors and **hilar (Leydig) cell tumors** are rare conditions in which the neoplasms secrete androgens. They can often be distinguished from each other in that Sertoli–Leydig tumors usually present in young women with palpable masses and hilar cell tumors are found in postmenopausal women with nonpalpable masses.

Granulosa–theca cell tumors and **gonadoblastomas** are other examples of androgen-secreting ovarian tumors.

Abnormal Uterine Bleeding

Definitions   180

Abnormal Premenopausal Bleeding   180

Postmenopausal Bleeding   181

Other Bleeding Tips   182

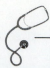

Menorrhagia: Bleeding too long or too much. Clinically signified by clots, anemia, increase in number of pads or tampons, and soiled clothing.

Metrorrhagia — the metro never comes according to schedule (bleeding at irregular intervals).

DEFINITIONS

Menstrual abnormalities include:

- **Polymenorrhea**: Menses with intervals that are too short (< 24 days).
- **Menorrhagia**: Menses that are too long in duration (> 7 days) and/or menses associated with excessive blood loss (> 80 mL) occurring at *regular* intervals.
- **Oligomenorrhea**: Menses with intervals that are too long (cycle lasts > 35 days).
- **Metrorrhagia**: Bleeding occurring at irregular intervals; intermenstrual bleeding.
- **Menometrorrhagia**: Combination of both menorrhagia and metrorrhagia; menses too long in duration or excessive blood loss + irregular bleeding intervals.
- **Kleine regnung**: Bleeding for 1–2 days during ovulation (scant).

ABNORMAL PREMENOPAUSAL BLEEDING

First, rule out pregnancy.

Anovulatory

Anovulation results in constant endometrial proliferation without progesterone-mediated maturation and shedding. Overgrown endometrium sheds continually and irregularly.

Causes

- Polycystic ovarian syndrome (PCOS)
- Obesity
- Hyperestrogenism
- Teenagers, perimenopause

Ovulatory

Usually menorrhagia and/or intermenstrual bleeding. Secondary to abnormal endometrial hemostasis for any reason.

Causes

- Structural abnormalities (fibroids, polyps, adenomyosis)
- Coagulopathy
- Neoplasm/cancer
- Adenomyosis
- Hypothyroidism
- Intrauterine device (IUD)/oral contraceptives (OCPs)
- Infections

Evaluation

History
Menstrual cycle charting.

Labs

- Pregnancy test
- Pap smear
- Basal body temperature (BBT) monitoring
- Midluteal progesterone level
- Ultrasonography
- Hemoglobin

Treatment

- Depends on the cause and/or ovulatory status
- First-line treatment:
    - Nonsteroidal anti-inflammatory drugs (NSAIDs) (tranexamic acid/ mefenamic acid)
    - Iron supplements
    - Hormones
    - Ablation/D&C (reduces fertility)
    - Myomectomy
    - Hysterectomy
- Acute moderate to severe bleeding:
    - High-dose estrogens, progestins, or both
    - D&C, endometrial ablation
- Chronic:
    - NSAIDs
    - OCPs, progesterone-releasing IUD
    - Danazol
    - Low-dose progestins
    - Endometrial ablation, hysterectomy

Tumors (benign and malignant) often present with menorrhagia or metrorrhagia.

POSTMENOPAUSAL BLEEDING

Postmenopausal bleeding is vaginal bleeding after 1 year without period.

Differential Diagnoses for Postmenopausal Bleeding

- Vaginal/endometrial atrophy (most common)
- Endometrial hyperplasia/cancer
- Cervical cancer
- Vulvar cancer
- Estrogen-secreting tumor
- Fibroids
- Anticoagulation
- Spontaneous cycle
- Infections (pelvic inflammatory disease [PID])
- Trauma

Studies

- **Endometrial biopsy and endocervical curettage** (because of the prevalence and danger of endometrial lesions)
- Pap smear for cervical dysplasia, neoplasia; swabs for infections

Postcoital bleeds suggest trauma, infections, or cervical cancer.

Always do an endometrial biopsy when encountering postmenopausal bleeding and for women > 40 years old with abnormal bleeding because of the strong possiblity of endometrial cancer or hyperplasia.

- Ultrasound
- Hysteroscopy and D&C
- +/− Computed tomography (CT)

OTHER BLEEDING TIPS

- Postcoital bleeding in pregnant woman: Consider placenta previa/abortion.
- Postcoital bleeding in nonpregnant woman: Consider cervical cancer.
- Postmenopausal bleeding: Consider endometrial cancer.
- Premenopausal bleeding: Consider PCOD.

HIGH-YIELD FACTS IN

Pelvic Pain

Chronic Pelvic Pain 184

Acute Pelvic Pain 185

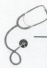

Pelvic pain accounts for 12% of hysterectomies, 20% of diagnostic laparoscopies, and 40% of repeat office visits.

Chronic pelvic pain: Think of "leapin' " pain.
Leiomyoma
Endometriosis
Adhesions, adenomyosis
Pelvic inflammatory disease (PID)
Infections other than PID
Neoplasia

PID is the most common cause of chronic pelvic pain in high-risk populations. Endometriosis is the most common cause in low-risk groups.

Mittelschmerz is pelvic pain associated with ovulation.

Definition and Criteria

- ≥ 6 months of pain
- Altered activities due to pain (e.g., missed work, homebound, depression, sexual dysfunction) or requires treatment
- Below the umbilicus

Etiologies

- Leiomyoma
- Endometriosis/adenomyosis
- Adhesions
- Pelvic inflammatory disease (PID)
- Infections other than PID
- Neoplasia
- Gastrointestinal (inflammatory bowel disease [IBD])
- Psychological/psychiatric
- Fibromyalgia
- Urinary tract infection (UTI)
- Ovulation

Workup

1. Detailed history (focusing on above etiologies):
   - Temporal pattern
   - Pain characteristics
   - Associated symptoms
   - Past surgeries
   - Last menstrual period (LMP)
   - GI complaints
2. Physical exam:

   Look for:
   - Masses
   - Cervical motion tenderness
   - Neurological testing
   - Bladder/urological etiology
   - Pelvic organ nodularity
   - Vulvar or pelvic floor tenderness
   - Anus
3. Relation of pain to basal body temperature elevation (to rule out mittelschmerz pain associated with ovulation).
4. Blood work:
   - Complete blood count (CBC)
   - Pregnancy test
   - STS (serotest for syphilis), VDRL (Venereal Disease Research Laboratory test), gonococcus, chlamydia
   - Urinalysis (UA)
   - Occult blood
5. Radiographic studies:
   - Abdominal and pelvic sonogram

For further evaluation:

- Computed tomography (CT)
- Magnetic resonance imaging (MRI)
- Barium enema
- Bone scan
- Renal sonogram/intravenous pyelogram (IVP)

6. Colonoscopy and/or cystoscopy (should be performed if all above are inconclusive).
7. Rule out psychosomatic pain.
8. Diagnostic laparoscopy.

Laparoscopy is the final, conclusive step in diagnosing pelvic pain, but it should only be done once psychogenic causes are considered carefully.

ACUTE PELVIC PAIN

Etiologies

- Gynecologic—may require surgery:
  - Ruptured ovarian cyst
  - Adnexal torsion
  - Tubo-ovarian abscess, PID
- Obstetric:
  - Ectopic pregnancy
  - Abortion
- GI/genitourinary (GU):
  - Diverticulitis
  - Appendicitis
  - UTI
  - IBD, irritable bowel syndrome (IBS)

Differential of acute pelvic pain:
"A ROPE"
- **A**ppendicitis
- **R**uptured ovarian cyst
- **O**varian torsion
- **P**ID (abscess)
- **E**ctopic pregnancy

Workup

1. History
2. Physical exam (cervical motion tenderness, adnexal tenderness, and abdominal tenderness are all signs of PID)
3. Labs:
   - Pregnancy test (positive might indicate ectopic pregnancy or abortion)
   - CBC (PID or appendicitis might give elevated WBCs)
   - UA (leukocytes indicate possible UTI)
4. Pelvic sonogram (will show cysts and torsion)
5. Diagnostic laparoscopy vs. laparotomy.

Ruptured cyst is the most common cause of acute pelvic pain.

Treatment

Based on cause of pain.

Endometriosis and Adenomyosis

Endometriosis   188

Adenomyosis   190

Adenomyosis vs. Endometriosis   190

Tissue in endometriosis is viable and behaves normally.

Exam scenario:
A 37-year-old woman complains of hemoptysis with each period.
Diagnosis: Endometriosis of nasopharynx or lung.

Severity of symptoms does not necessarily correlate with quantity of ectopic endometrial tissue.

Complications of endometriosis:
Prolonged bleeding causes scarring, which leads to adhesions.
Adhesions cause infertility and possibly small bowel obstructions.

Definition

The condition in which endometrial tissue is found outside of the uterus, often causing pain and/or infertility.

Incidence

- 10–15%.
- Accounts for 20% of chronic pelvic pain.
- One third of women affected with infertility have endometriosis.

Pathophysiology

The ectopic endometrial tissue is functional. It responds to hormones and goes through cyclic changes, such as menstrual bleeding.

The result of this ectopic tissue is "ectopic menses," which causes bleeding, peritoneal inflammation, pain, fibrosis, and, eventually, adhesions.

Sites of Endometriosis

Common
- Ovary (bilaterally)
- Cul-de-sac
- Fallopian tubes
- Uterosacral ligaments
- Bowel

Less Common
- Cervix
- Vagina
- Bladder

Rare
- Nasopharynx
- Lungs
- CNS
- Abdominal wall

Adhesions

Adhesions from prolonged endometriosis can cause:
- **Infertility** from fallopian tube or outer uterine adhesions
- **Small bowel obstruction** from intestinal adhesions
- **Pelvic pain**
- **Difficult operations** (laparoscopy/laparotomy)

Theories of Etiology

Though the etiology is unknown, there are four theories:

1. **Retrograde menstruation:** Endometrial tissue fragments are transported through the fallopian tubes and implant there or intra-abdominally.
2. **Mesothelial (peritoneal) metaplasia:** Peritoneal tissue becomes endometrial-like and responds to hormones.

3. **Vascular/lymphatic transport:** Endometrial tissue is transported via blood vessels and lymphatics.
4. **Altered immunity:** There may be deficient or inadequate natural killer (NK) or cell-mediated response.

Risk Factor

Family history.

Clinical Presentation

Most commonly in women in their late 20s and early 30s:
- Pelvic pain (worse during menses):
  - Dysmenorrhea
  - Dyspareunia—implants on pouch of Douglas
  - Dyschezia (pain with defecation)—implants on rectosigmoid
- Infertility
- Vaginal staining (from vaginal implants)

Dyspareunia (painful intercourse) presents most commonly as pain with deep penetration.

Signs

- Retroflexed, tender uterus.
- Nodular uterosacral ligaments.
- Ovarian mass (endometrioma): "Chocolate cyst"—an implant that occurs *within the ovarian capsule* and bleeds, creating a small blood-filled cavity in the ovary.
- Blue/brown vaginal implants (rare).

Diagnosis

1. **Laparoscopy or laparotomy:** Ectopic tissue *must be biopsied for diagnosis:*
   - Blue implants—new
   - Brown implants—older
   - White implants—oldest (scar tissue)
2. **Biopsy:** Positive findings contain glands, stroma, hemosiderin.

Maximum time on estrogen suppression should be 6 months due to adverse effects.

Clinical Course

- 30% asymptomatic.
- If left untreated, most lead to increasing pain and possible bowel complications.
- Often, there is improvement with pregnancy secondary to temporary cessation of menses.
- Associated with infertility.

Treatment

Medical (Temporizing)

- All of these treatments suppress estrogen:
  - GnRH agonists (leuprolide)—suppress follicle-stimulating hormone (FSH); creates a pseudomenopause.
  - Depo-Provera (progesterone [+/– estrogen])—creates a pseudopregnancy.
  - Danazol—an androgen derivative that suppresses FSH/LH, thus also causing pseudomenopause.

The pulsatile fashion of endogenous GnRH stimulates FSH secretion. GnRH agonists are not pulsatile and therefore suppress FSH.

GnRH is associated with osteoporosis; should be used for only 6 months.

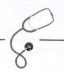

Pseudomenopause — ↓ FSH/LH rather than ↑ FSH/LH as seen in "real" menopause.

Dysmenorrhea in adenomyosis doesn't occur as cyclically as it does in endometriosis.

Endometrial ablation will not improve adenomyosis symptoms.

- Oral contraceptives (OCPs)—used with mild disease/symptoms.
  - Pseudopregnancy:
    - Nonsteroidal anti-inflammatory drugs (NSAIDs) for analgesia.
    - OCPs.
    - Medroxyprogesterone.

Surgical

- Conservative (if reproductivity is to be preserved): **Laparoscopic lysis** of adhesions and implants.
- Definitive: Total abdominal hysterectomy and bilateral salpingo-oophorectomy (TAH/BSO).

ADENOMYOSIS

Definition

Endometrial tissue found *within the myometrium,* resulting in a symmetrically enlarged and globular uterus.

Incidence

- 15%.
- Usually in parous women in their 30s and 40s. Rare in nulliparous women.
- Often coexists with uterine fibroids and to a lesser extent with endometriosis.

Signs and Symptoms

Common
- Uterine enlargement
- Dysmenorrhea
- Menorrhagia

Treatment

- GnRH agonist
- Mifepristone (RU 486)—a progesterone antagonist
- TAH if severe

ADENOMYOSIS VS. ENDOMETRIOSIS

Adenomyosis

- Found in older women
- Doesn't respond to hormonal stimulation
- Noncyclical

Endometriosis

- Found in young women
- Tissue is responsive to estrogen
- Cyclical

Pelvic Masses

Differential Diagnoses   192

Diagnostic Tests for Various Causes of Pelvic Masses   192

Functional Ovarian Cysts   193

Leiomyomas (Fibroids)   194

Leiomyomas are the most common causes of undiagnosed pelvic masses.

Pregnancy tests should be done in all women of reproductive age.

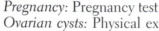

DIFFERENTIAL DIAGNOSES

- Functional cyst
- Pregnancy
- Infection/inflammation (tubo-ovarian abscess [TOA], diverticular abscess, appendicitis)
- Benign (fibroid, teratoma, ovarian cyst)
- Malignant (ovaries, fallopian tubes, colon, cervix, metastatic)

DIAGNOSTIC TESTS FOR VARIOUS CAUSES OF PELVIC MASSES

Pregnancy: Pregnancy test
Ovarian cysts: Physical exam (+ ultrasound [US] if needed for confirmation)
Leiomyoma: Physical exam (+ US, hysteroscopy if needed for confirmation)
Ovarian neoplasm: US, computed tomography (CT) scan, CA-125 level, surgical exploration, high level of suspicion due to age, family history
Endometrial neoplasm: Endocervical curettage, dilation and curettage (D&C)
Endometriosis/adenomyosis: Laparotomy/laparoscopy
TOA: History of pelvic inflammatory disease (PID), tender mass, nonspecific colon cancer (Figure 17-1)

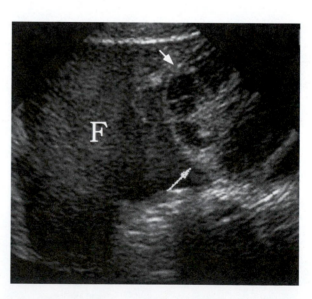

FIGURE 17-1. Tubo-ovarian abscess.

Endovaginal sonogram of a patient with pelvic pain, vaginal discharge, and fever. The sonogram demonstrates echogenic fluid (F) in the cul-de-sac and a large cystic mass with internal echoes (arrows) in the left adnexa. This patient was known to have pelvic inflammatory disease and was successfully treated with antibiotics. (Reproduced, with permission, from Tierney LM, McPhee SJ, Papadakis MA, eds. *Current Medical Diagnosis & Treatment 2006*. Gonzales R, Zeiger R, online eds. Photo courtesy of P Callen.)

Follicular Cysts

Follicular cysts are the most common functional ovarian cysts.

Physiology

Failure of rupture or incomplete resorption of the ovarian follicle results in a cyst. Just like the original follicle, the ovarian cyst is granulosa cell lined and contains a clear to yellow estrogen-rich fluid.

Signs and Symptoms

- Usually asymptomatic when small (< 5 cm). The larger the size, the more pain they cause and the higher the risk of torsion.
- Polymenorrhea/oligomenorrhea.
- Unilateral abdominal pain.
- Acute pelvic pain often signifies rupture.

DIAGNOSIS

- Physical exam—pelvic and abdominal exam.
- US confirms the diagnosis and is also helpful to see whether the cyst is ruptured.

TREATMENT

- No treatment is necessary for most cysts, since they usually resolve spontaneously within 2 months.
- Oral contraceptives (OCPs) may aid in the symptomatic patient.
- If the cyst is unresolved after 2 months, laparotomy/laparoscopy is indicated to evaluate/rule out neoplasia/endometriosis.
- Chronically symptomatic cysts can be managed with OCPs if no other underlying cause (e.g., neoplasia) is found.
- Surgical resection can be considered for symptomatic cysts > 5 cm.

Large ovarian cysts increase the risk of ovarian torsion, which is a medical emergency.

Lutein Cysts

There are two types of lutein cysts: **Corpus luteum cysts** and **theca lutein cysts.**

CORPUS LUTEUM CYST

The corpus luteum cyst is an enlarged and longer living, but *otherwise normal*, corpus luteum. It can produce progesterone for weeks longer than normal, delaying menses. **Corpus hemorragicum** is formed when there is hemorrhage into a corpus luteum cyst. If this ruptures, the patient will present with acute lower-quadrant pain and bleeding and may develop signs of shock and hemoperitoneum.

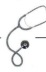

Pregnancy test must be performed to rule out ectopic pregnancy in all cases of pelvic pain and amenorrhea.

Signs and Symptoms

Unilateral tenderness + amenorrhea.

Amenorrhea in corpus luteum cysts is due to prolonged progesterone production.

HIGH-YIELD FACTS

Pelvic Masses

Diagnosis

History and pelvic exam, US.

Treatment

Only if symptomatic: Analgesics, OCPs, laparotomy/laparoscopy if ruptured.

THECA LUTEIN CYST

Increased levels of human chorionic gonadotropin (hCG) can cause *follicular overstimulation* and lead to theca lutein cysts, which are often multiple and bilateral.

Conditions that cause elevated hCG levels:
- Gestational trophoblastic disease (molar pregnancy)
- Polycystic ovarian disease
- Ovulation-inducing agents (clomiphene or hCG)
- Multiple gestation

LEIOMYOMAS (FIBROIDS)

Leiomyomas are localized, benign, *smooth muscle tumors* of the uterus. They are *hormonally responsive* and therefore become bigger and smaller corresponding to the menstrual cycle.

Epidemiology

- Clinically found in 25–33% of reproductive-age women and in up to 50% of black women.
- They are almost always multiple.
- The most common indication for hysterectomy.

Sequelae

Changes in uterine fibroids over time (i.e., postmenopausal) include:
- Hyaline degeneration
- Calcification
- Red degeneration (painful interstitial hemorrhage, often with pregnancy)
- Cystic degeneration—may rupture into adjacent cavities

Uterine Locations of Leiomyomas

Submucous—just below endometrium; tend to bleed
Intramural—within the uterine wall
Subserous—just below the serosa/peritoneum
Cervical—in the cervix

Symptoms

- **Asymptomatic** in > 50% of cases
- **Bleeding** +/– anemia—one third of cases present with bleeding. Bleeding is usually menorrhagia, caused by:
  - Abnormal blood supply
  - Pressure ulceration
  - Abnormal endometrial covering
- **Pain**—secondary dysmenorrhea
- **Pelvic pressure**
- **Infertility**

Diagnosis

- **Physical exam** (bimanual pelvic and abdominal exams): Fibroids are smooth, firm, and usually midline.

Extremely rarely do leiomyomas progress to malignancy (leiomyosarcoma).

Eighty percent of women have uterine fibroids on pathological evaluation.

Leiomyomas are most commonly of the subserous type.

Submucosal and intramural types of fibroids usually present as menorrhagia. Subserous type often presents with torsion.

- **Sonography** (may also be visualized by x-ray, magnetic resonance imaging [MRI], CT, hysterosalpingogram [HSG], hysteroscopy, or intravenous urogram)
- Pap, ECC, endometrial biopsy, hysteroscopy, and D&C can be done to rule out malignancy.

Treatment

- *No treatment* is indicated for most women, as this hormonally sensitive tumor will likely shrink with menopause/pregnancy/not menstruating.
- Pregnancy is usually *uncomplicated.* Bed rest and narcotics are indicated for pain with red degeneration.
- Treatment is usually initiated when:
  - Tumor is > 12–14 weeks' gestation size.
  - Hematocrit falls.
  - Tumor compresses adjacent structures.
  - Symptoms limit lifestyle.

Gonadotropin-releasing hormone (GnRH) agonists can be given for up to 6 months to shrink tumors (i.e., before surgery) and control bleeding:

- **Myomectomy**: Surgical removal of the fibroid in infertile patients with no other reason for infertility.
- **Hysterectomy**: Indicated for women without future reproductive plans and with unremitting disability.

Pregnancy with fibroids carries increased relative risk:
- Abruption   3.87
- First-trimester bleeding   1.82
- Dysfunctional labor   1.85
- Breech   3.98
- C-section   6.39

About one third of fibroids recur following myomectomy.

NOTES

Cervical Dysplasia

Overview	198
Risk Factors for Cervical Dysplasia and Cervical Cancer	198
Squamocolumnar Junction (SCJ)	198
Pap Smear	198
Colposcopy with Cervical Biopsy and ECC	201
Cone Biopsy and Leep	201
Cryotherapy	202
Laser Therapy	202

Squamous cell carcinoma of the cervix is almost nonexistent in women who have had no sexual contact.

Risk factors for cervical dysplasia: OSHA Ends Dirt, Garbage, and Chemicals:
Oral contraceptives
Sex
HPV
Alcohol
Education/poverty
Diethylstilbestrol (DES)
Genetics
Cigarettes

The adolescent cervix is more susceptible to carcinogenic stimuli.

OVERVIEW

Cervical dysplasia and cervical cancer lie on a continuum of conditions. Cervical dysplasia can take one of three paths:
1. Progress to cancer
2. Remain the same and not progress
3. Regress to normal

RISK FACTORS FOR CERVICAL DYSPLASIA AND CERVICAL CANCER

- Human papillomavirus (HPV) infection:
  - 80% of cases
  - Risk highest if infected > 6 months
  - Types 16, 18, 31, 33, 45—high oncogenic potential
- High sexual activity (increase risk of viral/bacterial infections):
  - Multiple sexual partners
  - Intercourse at early age (≤ 17 years)
- Low socioeconomic status.
- Genetic predisposition.
- Cigarette smoking (cocarcinogen substances).
- Alcohol, 2–4 drinks/wk, can increase risk of HPV infection.
- Oral contraceptives (OCPs), particularly with use > 5 years (condoms decrease risk in these women).
- Young women whose mothers took diethylstilbestrol (DES) during pregnancy.
- Immunodeficiency.

SQUAMOCOLUMNAR JUNCTION (SCJ)

- Most cervical cancers arise at this site.
- Position is variable (see Figure 19-1):
  - In nulliparous women it is usually located at the external cervical os.
  - After pregnancy it migrates out and is visible to the naked eye (*endocervical ectropion*).
  - Ectropions become reepithelialized by squamous epithelium and become the *transformation zone*.
- The transformation or the SCJ must be biopsied to rule out cancer or precancer.

PAP SMEAR

A cytologic screening test for cervical neoplasia.

Technique

- A speculum is placed in the vagina to expose the uterine cervix (no digital exams or lubricants in the vagina prior to the Pap).
- Cells are scraped from the ectocervix with a spatula, then from the endocervix using an endocervical brush.

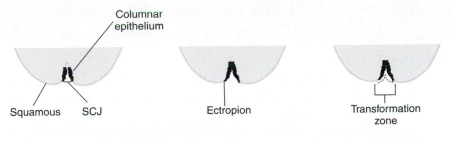

Columnar epithelium

Squamous   SCJ

Ectropion

Transformation zone

FIGURE 19-1. Sites of cervical cancers.

- The cells are smeared on a glass slide, fixative spray is applied, and the cells are examined.
- New technique: Cervix is scraped and swabbed as above, but the sample is placed in liquid medium (Thin Prep).

Success Rate

- Decreases incidence and mortality rate of invasive cervical cancer by 90%
- 80% sensitivity
- 90% specificity

Indications

According to the American College of Obstetricians and Gynecologists (ACOG) (2003) recommendations:

- "Routine annual screening should begin 3 years after the initiation of sexual activity but no later than 21" (ACOG, 2003).
- If three consecutive Pap smears and pelvic exams 1 year apart are normal in women ≥ 30 years old who have no risk factors, the screening interval can be lengthened (average 2–3 years).
- Lengthening of interval is not recommended if the patient or her sexual partner has more than one other sexual partner.

Microscopic Analysis

Cytologic analysis of cells taken from a Pap smear will indicate cervical dysplasia if there is:

- Clumping of chromatin
- Decreased cytoplasm resulting in a higher nucleus/cytoplasm ratio

Classification of Abnormalities

Remember, Pap smear gives information about cervical cytology. Two different systems exist that describe the possible findings of a Pap smear:

1. Modern classification system (cervical intraepithelial neoplasia [CIN]): Describes the degree of abnormality of the cells.
2. Bethesda staging system (squamous intraepithelial lesion [SIL]): Describes three things: (1) the adequacy of the Pap test performed, (2) the degree of abnormality, and (3) a description of the cells.

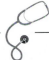

Cervical dysplasia almost always forms at transformation zone or squamocolumnar junction (SCJ).

Two things to remember about Pap smear:
1. It is a screening tool.
2. It provides cytologic information, not histologic.

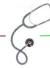

Are the results of a Pap enough to diagnose cervical cancer? No—Pap smear only gives cytology. Colposcopy and biopsy are needed for histology, which is necessary for diagnosis, staging, and treatment.

Table 19-1 correlates the Bethesda staging with the CIN staging. All the terms are possible results of a Pap smear.

Findings and Workup

- Atypical squamous cells of undetermined significance (ASCUS): Repeat Pap every 4–6 months until three consecutive negative smears or HPV testing +/– colposcopy.
- Atypical glandular cells of undetermined significance (AGCUS): Colposcopy and endometrial sampling + endocervical curettage.
- Low-grade squamous intraepithelial lesion (LGSIL): Colposcopy with endocervical curettage (ECC) and biopsies.
- High-grade squamous intraepithelial lesion (HGSIL): Colposcopy with ECC.

Very complex, many algorithms. Protocols available online at www.asccp.org.

TABLE 19-1. Modern Classification System vs. Bethesda Staging System

	MODERN CLASSIFICATION SYSTEM (CIN)	BETHESDA STAGING
Squamous lesions	Normal	Normal Benign cellular changes
	Atypical cells, possible inflammatory	Reactive cellular changes Atypical squamous cells of undetermined significance (ASCUS)
	CIN I—mild dysplasia: Neoplastic cells confined to lower one third of epithelium (60% spontaneously regress)	Low-grade squamous intraepithelial lesion (LGSIL)
	CIN II—moderate dysplasia: Involvement of two thirds of epithelium (43% regress)	High-grade squamous intraepithelial lesion (HGSIL)
	CIN III—severe dysplasia (carcinoma in situ): Involvement up to the basement membrane of the epithelium (33% regress, 12% advance to invasive cancer)	
	Squamous cell carcinoma	Squamous cell carcinoma
Glandular lesions	Atypical glandular cells	Atypical glandular cells of undetermined significance (AGCUS) AGCUS divides into endocervical or endometrial

Definition

Low-magnification microscopic viewing of cervix, vagina, and vulva. Provides illuminated, magnified view, which aids in identifying lesions.

Indications

- ASCUS with high-risk HPV subtypes
- ASCUS suggestive of high-grade lesion (ASC-H)
- Atypical glandular cells (AGUS)
- LGSIL
- HGSIL

Procedure

1. Speculum is inserted for visualization of the cervix.
2. Acetic acid is applied. Acetic acid dehydrates cells and causes precipitation of nucleic proteins in the superficial layers. The neoplastic cells appear whiter because of higher nucleus/cytoplasm ratio.
3. Colposcopy: Then a low-power microscope (colposcope) is used to look for dysplasia. Signs of dysplasia include whiteness and abnormal vessels.
4. Cervical biopsy: Neoplastic and dysplastic areas are then biopsied under colposcopic guidance. Contraindications include acute PID or cervicitis. Pregnancy is NOT a contraindication.
5. ECC: A curette is then placed in the cervical canal to obtain endocervical cells for cytologic examination.

Ninety percent of women with abnormal cytologic findings can be adequately evaluated with colposcopy.

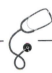

What must be completely visualized for adequate colposcopic evaluation? The transformation zone.

Information Provided by Colposcopy and ECC

If biopsy results or ECC is positive for CIN II or III, cone biopsy or loop electrodiathermy excision procedure (LEEP).

Cone biopsy: A procedure performed in the operating room in which a cone-shaped biopsy is removed, including part of the endocervical canal.
LEEP: A procedure performed in an office setting in which a small wire loop can be electrified to cauterize and remove a biopsy sample: Part of the endocervical canal is removed.

Indications for Cone Biopsy/LEEP

1. Inadequate view of transformation zone on colposcopy.
2. Positive ECC.
3. ± 2 grade discrepancy between colposcopic biopsy and Pap.
4. Treatment for HGSIL.
5. Treatment for adenocarcinoma-in-situ.
6. When cancer cannot be excluded after colposcopy, biopsy, and ECC.

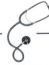

Evaluation of biopsy margins may be difficult with LEEP.

HIGH-YIELD FACTS

Cervical Dysplasia

LEEP as Treatment

LEEP can also be used to diagnose and treat CIN and VIN (vulvar intraep-ithelial neoplasia).

Guidelines for LEEP Treatment
- Never treat during pregnancy.
- Never treat without excluding invasive carcinoma.
- When treating, ablate entire transformation zone.
- Always excise keratinizing lesions.

CRYOTHERAPY

An outpatient procedure that uses a probe cooled with N_2O to $-70°F$ to ablate lesions.

Indications

Treatment of LGSIL or HGSIL only if it is a lesion completely visualized on colposcopic exam.

Complications

Discharge, failure of therapy for HGSIL.

LASER THERAPY

Light Amplification by Stimulated Emission of Radiation (LASER): A high-energy photon beam generates heat at impact and vaporizes tissue.

Indications

1. Excision or ablation of CIN
2. Ablation during laparoscopic surgery (e.g., endometriosis)

Cervical Cancer

Epidemiology	204
Symptoms	204
Differential Diagnosis	204
Types of Cervical Cancer	204
Sites of Distant Organ Metastases (in Order of Frequency)	205
Clinical Staging of Invasive Cervical Cancer	205
Treatment of Invasive Cervical Cancer	205
Treatment for Bulky Central Pelvic Disease	208
Recurrent Cervical Carcinoma	208
Clear Cell Adenocarcinoma of Cervix and Vagina	210

Age Affected

- Peak incidence between ages 45 and 55.
- Fifteen percent of women develop it before age 30.
- Increasing percentage of women diagnosed before 20 years of age (perhaps due to early screening or changes in sexual patterns).

Race Prevalence

- More prevalent in African-American women and urban Hispanic women than white women.
- African-American mortality rate is two times greater than whites.

SYMPTOMS

Symptoms of cervical cancer become evident when cervical lesions are of moderate size.

Early Stages
- None
- Irregular/prolonged vaginal bleeding/pink discharge
- Postcoital bleeding (brownish discharge)

Middle Stages
- Postvoid bleeding
- Dysuria/hematuria

Advanced Stages
- Weight loss
- Bloody, malodorous discharge
- Severe pain, due to spread to sacral plexus

DIFFERENTIAL DIAGNOSIS

- Eversions
- Polyps, nabothian cysts
- Papillary endocervicitis/papillomas/inflammation
- Vaginal malignancies

Tuberculosis, syphilitic chancres, and granuloma inguinale can also cause cervical lesions.

TYPES OF CERVICAL CANCER

Cancer cells create foci of keratinization with cornified "pearls" that can be visible.

Squamous Cell Cancer

Accounts for **80% of cervical cancer.**

Types

- Keratinizing
- Nonkeratinizing: *Well-demarcated* tumor–stromal borders

- Small-cell carcinoma: Small, round, or spindle-shaped cell with *poorly defined* tumor–stromal borders

Adenocarcinoma

- Accounts for **10–20%** of all invasive cervical cancers.
- Arises from columnar cells lining the endocervical canal and glands.
- **Early diagnosis is difficult; the false-negative rate with Pap smear is 80%.**

Cancers Metastatic to Cervix by Direct Extension

- **R**ectal
- **I**ntra-abdominal
- **B**ladder
- **E**ndometrial

Occasionally (via hematogenous spread): Breast, lung

Adenocarcinoma is relatively resistant to radio- and chemotherapy compared to squamous cell carcinoma.

Cancers that metastasize to cervix:
Remember: **RIB E**ye steak.
Rectal
Intra-abdominal
Bladder
Endometrial

SITES OF DISTANT ORGAN METASTASES (IN ORDER OF FREQUENCY)

1. Lung
2. Liver
3. Bone

CLINICAL STAGING OF INVASIVE CERVICAL CANCER

Clinical staging of cervical cancer is important for prognosis and treatment (see Tables 20-1 through 20-4).

Modes of Staging

- Pelvic and rectal exam (under anesthesia).
- Chest x-ray.
- Liver function tests.
- Evaluate genitourinary tract via intravenous pyelogram or computed tomography (CT) with intravenous contrast dye.
- Evaluate lymph node enlargements or abnormalities with external CT-guided biopsies.
- Intraoperative evaluation may help.

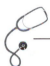

Cervical cancer is staged clinically.

TREATMENT OF INVASIVE CERVICAL CANCER

- **Radical surgery**: Radical hysterectomy with lymph node dissection.
- **Radiation therapy**: High-dose delivery to the cervix and vagina, and minimal dosing to the bladder and rectum:
  - External beam whole pelvic radiation.
  - Transvaginal intracavitary cesium—transvaginal applicators allow significantly larger doses of radiation to surface of cervix.

Radical hysterectomy requires removal of:
- Uterus
- Cervix
- Parametrial tissue
- Upper vagina
+ Pelvic lymphadenectomy from the bifurcation of the aorta to the level of the inguinal ligament.

TABLE 20-1. Staging of Invasive Cervical Cancer

INTERNATIONAL FEDERATION OF GYNECOLOGISTS AND OBSTETRICIANS (FIGO) STAGE	DESCRIPTION OF CARCINOMA	5-YEAR SURVIVAL RATE POST TREATMENT
0	In situ; intraepithelial carcinoma	
I	Confined to cervix; preclinical IA Preclinical (Diagnosis only by microscopy) ■ Minimal microscopic invasion of stroma: ■ Max of 7-mm horizontal spread and 5-mm stromal invasion	65–90%
	IA-1 ≤ 3-mm depth	≈ 94%
	IA-2 > 3-mm to ≤ 5-mm depth of stromal invasion	≈ 92%
	IB ■ Clinically confined to cervix ■ Preclinical greater than IA-2	85%
	IB-1 Clinical lesion ≤ 4 cm in diameter	90%
	IB-2 Lesion > 4 cm in diameter	79%
II	■ Carcinoma extends beyond cervix ■ Has not extended to pelvic wall ■ Involves upper two thirds of vagina, but not lower third	45–80% 30–40% if adenocarcinoma
	IIA No parametrial involvement	≈ 76%
	IIB Obvious parametrial involvement	≈ 73%
III	■ Carcinoma extended to pelvic wall ■ No cancer-free space between the tumor and the pelvic wall (on rectal exam) ■ Tumor involves lower one third of vagina ■ Hydronephrosis or nonfunctioning kidney	< 60% 20–30% if adenocarcinoma
	IIIA Does not involve pelvic wall	≈ 50%
	IIIB Involves pelvic wall	≈ 46%
IV	Carcinoma extends beyond true pelvis or Clinically involves mucosa of bladder or rectum	< 15%
	IVA Spread to adjacent organs	≈ 29%
	IVB Spread to distant organs	≈ 22%

TABLE 20-2. TNM Category Staging

T		FIRST RESECTION OF PRIMARY TUMOR
	TX	Primary tumor cannot be assessed.
	T0	No evidence of primary tumor.
	T1	Confined to cervix.
	T2	Beyond cervix. Upper two thirds of vagina but not lower one third.
	T2a	No parametrium.
	T2b	Parametrial involvement.
	T3	Tumor extends to pelvic wall. Involves lower one third of vagina. Kidney dysfunction.
	T3a	Pelvic wall not involved.
	T3b	Pelvic wall involved.
	T4	Distant metastasis.
	T4a	Adjacent organs.
	T4b	Distant organs.
Tis	0	Carcinoma in situ.
T1	I	Cervical carcinoma confined to uterus (extension to corpus should be disregarded).
T1a	IA	Invasive carcinoma diagnosed only by microscopy. All macroscopically visible lesions—even with superficial invasion—are T1b/IB. Stromal invasion with a maximal depth of 5.0 mm measured from the base of the epithelium and a horizontal spread of 7.0 mm. Vascular space involvement, venous or lymphatic, does not affect classification.
T1a1	IA1	Measured stromal invasion ≤ 3 mm in depth and ≤ 7 mm in lateral spread.
T1a2	IA2	Measured stromal invasion > 3.00 mm and ≤ 5.0 mm with a horizontal spread ≤ 7.0.
T1b	IB	Clinically visible lesion confined to the cervix or microscopic lesion > IA2.
T1b1	IB1	Clinically visible lesion ≤ 4.0 in greatest dimension.
	IB2	Clinically visible lesion > 4.0 cm.

TABLE 20-2. TNM Category Staging (continued)

N		REGIONAL LYMPH NODES
	NX	Regional lymph nodes cannot be assessed.
	N0	No regional lymph node metastasis.
	N1	Regional lymph node metastasis.
M		**DISTANT METASTASIS**
	MX	Presence of distant metastasis cannot be assessed.
	M0	No distant metastasis.
	M1	Distant metastasis (excludes peritoneal metastasis).

Used with the permission of the American Joint Committee on Cancer (AJCC), Chicago, Illinois. The original source for this material is the *AJCC Cancer Staging Manual,* Sixth Edition (2002), published by Springer-Verlag New York, Inc.

TREATMENT FOR BULKY CENTRAL PELVIC DISEASE

- Radical hysterectomy with adjuvant or neoadjuvant radiation therapy.
- Tumor cytoreduction: Use of cytotoxic chemotherapy before definitive treatment with radiation or radical surgery.

RECURRENT CERVICAL CARCINOMA

Recurs within 2–3 years of primary treatment.

TABLE 20-3. Grading of Cervical Carcinoma

GRADE	INVASIVE SQUAMOUS TUMOR	ADENOCARCINOMA
X	Cannot be assessed	
1	Well differentiated	■ Small component of solid growth and nuclear atypia ■ Mild to moderate
2	Moderately differentiated	Intermediate-grade differentiation
3	Poorly differentiated	■ Solid pattern ■ Severe nuclear atypia predominate
4	Undifferentiated	

TABLE 20-4. Correlation of FIGO Stage with AJCC TNM Grouping

Stage 0	Tis	N0	M0
Stage IA1	T1a1	N0	M0
Stage IA2	T1a2	N0	M0
Stage IB1	T1b1	N0	M0
Stage IB2	T1b2	N0	M0
Stage IIA	T2a	N0	M0
Stage IIB	T2b	N0	M0
Stage IIIA	T3a	N0	M0
Stage IIIB	T3b	Any N	M0
Stage IVA	T4	Any N	M0
Stage IVB	Any T	Any N	M1

Screening

Look for:
- Vaginal bleeding
- Hematuria/dysuria
- Constipation/melena
- Pelvic and leg pain
- Fistulas
- Sacral backache or pain in sciatic distribution
- Costovertebral angle and flank pain

Cause of Death

Uremia and pyelonephritis are major causes of death in cervical cancer (found in 50% of patients). **Excretory urogram** can identify periureteral compression by tumor.

Treatment

- Patients may only be treated for cure if disease is confined to pelvis.
- Patients with central recurrence after radical hysterectomy are treated with **radiation.**
- Patients previously treated with radiotherapy are only treated by **radical pelvic surgery.**

- **Chemotherapy:**
  - Response rates higher with combination therapy.
  - Most combinations include platinum.
  - Response rates = 50–70% for 4–6 months of life.

CLEAR CELL ADENOCARCINOMA OF CERVIX AND VAGINA

Women who took DES during pregnancy have a 1.35% increased relative risk of breast cancer.

- Incidence in women exposed in utero to diethylstilbestrol (DES) = 1:1000
- Affects women aged 16–27; median age = 19 years
- Overall survival rate: 80%
- 5-year survival rate for stage I disease: > 90%

Screening of DES-Exposed Women

- Annual Pap smear
- Careful palpation of vaginal walls to rule out adenosis or masses

Treatment

- Similar to treatment of squamous cell carcinoma of cervix.
- Preferred treatment is radical hysterectomy and pelvic lymph node dissection for stage I or IIA.
- Vaginectomy if vagina is involved.

Disease Recurrence

- Most DES-related clear cell carcinomas recur ≤ 3 years of initial treatment.
- Pulmonary and supraclavicular nodal metastasis common → yearly screening chest x-ray recommended.

Endometrial Cancer

General Facts	212
Clinical Presentation	212
Differential Diagnosis of Postmenopausal Bleeding	212
Endometrial Hyperplasia	213
Workup for Endometrial Cancer	213
Staging of Endometrial Cancer	214
Grading	214
Treatment	215
Uterine Sarcoma	215

GENERAL FACTS

Type I (Most Common)

- An **estrogen-dependent neoplasm** that begins as proliferation of normal tissue: Over time, chronic proliferation becomes hyperplasia (abnormal tissue) and, eventually, neoplasia.
- Endometrial cancer is the most common gynecologic cancer. Most cases (> 75%) are diagnosed in *postmenopausal* women.

Type II

Unrelated to estrogen or hyperplasia. Tends to present with higher-grade or more aggressive tumors.

CLINICAL PRESENTATION

Abnormal bleeding is present in 90% of cases:

- Bleeding in postmenopausal women (classic)
  or
- Meno/metrorrhagia (in premenopausal cases)
  or
- Abnormal Pap smear: 1–5% of cases

Pap smears are *not* diagnostic, but a finding of abnormal glandular cells of unknown significance (AGCUS) leads to further investigation.

DIFFERENTIAL DIAGNOSIS OF POSTMENOPAUSAL BLEEDING

- Exogenous estrogens
- Atrophic endometritis/vaginitis
- Endometrial cancer
- Endometrial/cervical polyps
- Coagulopathy

Etiologies of Endometrial Cancer

- Ovarian failure (i.e., polycystic ovarian syndrome [PCOS])
- Exogenous estrogens
- Estrogen-producing tumors (i.e., granulosa cell tumors)
- Liver disease (a healthy liver metabolizes estrogen)
- Previous radiation (leading to sarcomas)

Risk Factors

- Obesity
- Early menarche/late menopause
- Nulliparity (not by itself; most likely when associated with anovulation)
- PCOS
- Diabetes mellitus
- Hypertension
- Endometrial hyperplasia

- Tamoxifen treatment for breast cancer (increases risk two to three times)
- Unopposed estrogen stimulation
- Familial predisposition

Protective Factors
- Combined oral contraceptives
- Cigarette smoking
- Multiparity

Diagnosis of Endometrial Hyperplasia and Cancer
- **Biopsy** (gold standard)
- Pap smear (to evaluate cervical involvement)
- Endocervical curettage (specimens from endocervix and cervix must be examined separately to determine if there has been spread)
- Ultrasound

A positive finding would include endometrial hyperplasia or cancer.

Any agent/behavior that lowers the level or time of exposure to estrogen decreases the risk of endometrial cancer.

ENDOMETRIAL HYPERPLASIA

Endometrial hyperplasia is a precancerous condition. Types include the following:

Simple (Cystic Hyperplasia without Atypia)
- *Glandular and stromal proliferation:* 1–2% progress to cancer (this is the most differentiated and lowest risk of cancer)

Complex (Adenomatous Hyperplasia without Atypia)
- *Only glandular proliferation* (both simple and complex are treated with progesterone)

Atypical
- Simple type of atypical
- Complex type of atypical
- Proliferation with **cytologic atypia**

Twenty-nine percent of atypical endometrial hyperplasias progress to cancer:
- Simple type is treated by hysterectomy.
- Complex type is treated like cancer.

In general, the most differentiated hyperplasia has the lowest risk of developing into cancer, and the least differentiated has the highest risk.

WORKUP FOR ENDOMETRIAL CANCER

After diagnosis of endometrial cancer is made, the following should be performed to evaluate for possible metastasis:
- Physical exam
- Pathology
- Chest x-ray
- Labs
- CA-125
- Abdominal and pelvic computed tomography (CT)

Histologic Subtypes

- **Endometroid** (ciliated adenocarcinoma)—75–80%
- **Papillary serous:**
  - *Poor prognosis*
  - No history of elevated estrogen
  - More common in blacks
  - Acts like ovarian cancer
  - Presents late (stage IV)
- **Sarcomas** (covered below)

STAGING OF ENDOMETRIAL CANCER

Staging is determined by the **extent of the tumor.** Therefore, **staging must be accomplished surgically,** not clinically, so the tumor can be visualized. This is always the first step in treatment (see Table 21-1).

GRADING

Grade is the most important prognostic indicator in endometrial cancer.

Grading is determined by the tumor **histology:**

GI   Well differentiated: < 5% solid pattern

GII   Moderately differentiated: 5–50% solid pattern

GIII Poorly differentiated: > 50% solid pattern

TABLE 21-1. Staging of Endometrial Cancer

STAGE	DESCRIPTION	5-YEAR SURVIVAL RATE POST TREATMENT
I: Only uterine involvement	IA: Limited to endometrium IB: Invasion < one half of myometrium IC: Invasion > one half of myometrium	90%
II: Cervical involvement	IIA: Endocervical glands only IIB: Invasion of cervical stroma	70%
III: Local spread	IIIA: Invasion of serosa and/or adnexa, and/or positive peritoneal cytology IIIB: Invasion of vagina IIIC: Mets to pelvic/para-aortic lymph nodes	50–60%
IV: Distant spread	IVA: Invasion of bladder and/or bowel IVB: Distant invasion, including intra-abdominal and/or inguinal lymph nodes	20%

Basic treatment for all stages (surgical staging is always the first step):

- Total abdominal hysterectomy (TAH)
- Bilateral salpingo-oophorectomy (BSO)
- +/– Nodal sampling
- Peritoneal washings

Adjuvant Therapy

After the above steps in treatment, adjuvant therapy depends on the stage.

Stages I–II **Adjuvant radiation therapy**

Stages III–IV **External beam radiation**
Hormone therapy: Progestin therapy is often used as adjuvant hormonal therapy:
- If the cancer is progesterone receptor positive—70% have a 5-year survival.
- If the cancer is progesterone receptor negative—15–20% have a 5-year survival.

Adjuvant chemotherapy
- Doxorubicin
- Cisplatin
- Carboplatin and paclitaxel

Side effects:
Doxorubicin: cardiotoxicity
Cisplatin: nephrotoxicity

Uterine sarcoma is classified separately from endometrial cancer:

- Rare form of uterine cancer
- Presents as a rapidly enlarging mass with bleeding
- Not from fibroids (< 1% of fibroids progress to cancer)
- Poor prognosis

Most cases are diagnosed with exploratory surgery for what was thought to be a uterine myoma (fibroid).

Types

- Leiomyosarcoma (LMS)
- Mixed mesodermal (MMD) (mixed müllerian sarcomas)
- Endometrial stromal sarcoma (ESS)

Diagnosis

- ≥ 10 mitosis/high-power field
- Usually diagnosed from specimen sent after hysterectomy
- Staged just like endometrial cancer

Treatment

- Surgical (TAH/BSO, nodes, washings)
- Plus adjuvant only if high risk of recurrence
  - Radiation may enhance local control after surgery. Unknown survival benefit.
  - Adjuvant chemotherapy has no role.

Ovarian Cancer

Epidemiology	218
Epithelial Cell Ovarian Cancer	218
Hereditary Ovarian Cancer Syndromes	219
Ovarian Cancer Workup	219
Staging	219
Treatment	220
Nonepithelial Ovarian Cancer	221
Fallopian Cell Carcinoma	223

There are two basic histologic types of ovarian cancer:
- Epithelial
- Nonepithelial

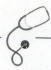

Ovarian cancer is the deadliest gynecologic cancer because it is difficult to detect before dissemination. It is the second most common gynecologic cancer.

70% of cases of ovarian cancer are diagnosed at stage III or IV.

Epithelial cell ovarian cancer accounts for 90% of all ovarian cancers.

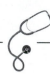

The serous type of epithelial ovarian cancer is the most common type of ovarian cancer and is bilateral 65% of the time.

A postmenopausal woman with widening girth notices that she can no longer button her pants.
Diagnosis: Ovarian cancer.

EPIDEMIOLOGY

- Second most common gynecologic malignancy.
- Fifth most common cancer for women.
- The deadliest gynecologic malignancy.
- Seventy percent of patients are diagnosed as stage III or IV.
- Lifetime risk is 1 in 70.

EPITHELIAL CELL OVARIAN CANCER

Ovarian cancer usually refers to epithelial cell type.

Histologic Subtypes

Five subtypes arising from epithelial tissue:
- Serous   75%
- Endometrioid   10%
- Mucinous   10%
- Undifferentiated   5%
- Clear cell   5%

Typical Clinical Presentation

Initial stages are usually asymptomatic. Signs/symptoms are usually from metastasis. Ovarian cancer typically spreads by exfoliation of cancerous cells into the peritoneal fluid. The peritoneal fluid carries it to other structures in the abdomen.

Signs and Symptoms

- Pelvic mass/pain
- Abdominal mass ("omental caking") (widening abdominal girth)
- Pleural effusion (dyspnea)
- Ascites
- Ventral hernia (due to increased intra-abdominal pressure)

CA-125

CA-125 is a tumor marker elevated in 80% of cases. It is useful in tracking the progression of the disease and the response to treatment.

Risk Factors

- Caucasian race
- Advanced age
- Family history
- Nulligravity

- Talc powder, high-fat diet, fertility drugs (data inconclusive on these)
- Early menarche, late menopause

Protective Factors

- Prolonged breast-feeding
- Oral contraceptives
- Multiparity
- Reproductive surgery/tubal ligation

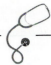

Omental caking is a fixed pelvic and upper abdominal mass with ascites. It is nearly pathognomonic for ovarian cancer.

HEREDITARY OVARIAN CANCER SYNDROMES

Five to ten percent of cases occur in association with genetically predisposed syndromes called **hereditary ovarian cancer (HOC) syndromes**. There are three types:

1. **Breast–ovarian cancer syndrome:** Involves cancer of the breast and ovary and is linked to the BRCA-1 and BRCA-2 genes in 90% of HOC.
2. **Lynch II syndrome—hereditary nonpolyposis colon cancer (HNPCC):** Involves sites that may include breast, ovaries, uterus, and colon.
3. **Site-specific ovarian cancer:** Accounts for < 1% and has an extremely strong genetic link. Usually, two or more first-degree relatives have the disease.

Ovarian cancer spread is normally through the peritoneal fluid, which carries cancer cells to other abdominal structures.

OVARIAN CANCER WORKUP

1. As with any pelvic mass, the first step of evaluation is ultrasound.
2. Definitive identification of adnexal mass by laparoscopy/laparotomy follows.

Ovarian cancer metastasis to the umbilicus is "Sister Mary Joseph's nodule."

Screening Recommendations

- Women with **standard risk** (fewer than two first-degree relatives with ovarian cancer): No routine screening recommended.
- Women with **high risk** (two or more first-degree relatives with ovarian cancer): Genetic testing and counseling.

If high risk, perform:
- Annual CA-125 (poor tool for screening).
- Annual transvaginal ultrasound.
- Annual pelvic exam.
- Consider BRCA screening. Consider prophylactic oophorectomy if positive.

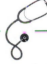

Large ovarian tumors can cause bowel obstruction and other GI symptoms.

STAGING

Ovarian cancer is staged surgically, not clinically (see Table 22-1).

About 25% of ovarian cancers occur in association with endometriosis.

Krukenberg's tumors are ovarian tumors that are metastatic from another primary cancer, usually from the gastrointestinal tract.

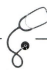

CA-125 is elevated in 80% of cases of ovarian cancer, but only in 50% of stage I cases. It is most useful as a tool to gauge progression/ regression of disease.

Ovarian and endometrial tumors are staged surgically, whereas cervical cancer is staged clinically.

TABLE 22-1. Staging of Ovarian Cancer

STAGE	DESCRIPTION	5-YEAR SURVIVAL RATE POST TREATMENT
I: Tumor limited to ovaries	IA: One ovary, capsule intact IB: Both ovaries, capsules intact IC: Tumor on ovary surface, capsule ruptured, ascites with malignant cells, or positive peritoneal washings	> 90%
II: Pelvic spread	IIA: Involvement of uterus/tubes IIB: Involvement of other pelvic structures IIC: IIA or IIB plus tumor on ovary surface, capsule ruptures, ascites with malignant cells, or positive peritoneal washings	70%
III: Spread to the abdominal cavity	IIIA: Positive abdominal peritoneal washings IIIB: < 2-cm implants on abdominal peritoneal surface IIIC: > 2-cm implants on abdominal peritoneal surface and/or positive retroperitoneal or inguinal nodes	25%
IV: Distant metastasis	Parenchymal liver/spleen spread Pleural effusion, skin or supraclavicular nodes	5%

TREATMENT

Surgery is used to get rid of as much of the tumor as possible, as well as to biopsy likely sites of spread. This always includes total abdominal hysterectomy/bilateral salpingo-oophorectomy and often includes lymph node sampling, omentectomy, and bladder and bowel resection. Debulking is the attempt to remove as much of the primary and metastatic tumor sites as possible and is employed in advanced disease.

Postop Management

First-line chemotherapy: Paclitaxel and cisplatin *or* paclitaxel and carboplatin:

Stage I–II   **Only chemotherapy** if stage IC/II or high-grade tumor

Stage III–IV **Chemotherapy,** plus:
Interval debulking if tumor > 2 cm (interval debulking means additional surgery after chemotherapy)

Poor Prognostic Indicators

- Short disease-free interval
- *Mucinous or clear cell tumor*
- Multiple disease sites
- *High/rising CA-125*

NONEPITHELIAL OVARIAN CANCER

Account for roughly 10–20% of ovarian cancers.

Histologic Types

- Germ cell: 8% of all ovarian cancers; include teratomas, dysgerminomas, choriocarcinomas.
- Gonadal–stromal: 1% of all ovarian cancers; include granulosa–theca cell tumors, Sertoli–Leydig tumors.

OVARIAN GERM CELL TUMORS (GCTs)

Eight percent of ovarian cancers are GCTs. They arise from totipotential germ cells that normally are able to differentiate into the three germ cell tissues. Ninety-five percent are benign.

Clinical Presentation

- Abdominal pain with rapidly enlarging palpable pelvic/abdominal mass
- Acute abdomen
- Fever
- Vaginal bleeding
- Usually found in children or young women

Types of Ovarian GCTs

Dysgerminoma

- Most common; arises from totally undifferentiated totipotential germ cells).
- Affects women **in teens to early 20s.**
- 20% bilateral.
- 20% associated with pregnancy.
- **LDH is the tumor marker** (see Table 22-2).

Endodermal Sinus Tumor

- Arises from extraembryonic tissues (yolk sac tumors).
- 20% of GCTs.
- Most aggressive GCT.
- Characteristic **Schiller–Duval bodies.**
- AFP is the tumor marker (see Table 22-2).

Signs and symptoms of GCTs are from the primary tumor, not mets (unlike epithelial ovarian cancer).

Teratoma

- Immature (malignant teratoma, teratoblastoma): Haphazard tissue from the ectoderm, mesoderm, and endoderm.
- Mature solid: Benign, unilateral.
- Mature cystic:
  - 95% of teratomas.
  - May contain hair, teeth, skin, sebum.
- Benign: Can lead to torsion.
- Struma ovarii:
  - Benign teratoma.
  - Mostly thyroid tissue.
  - May lead to hyperthyroidism.
- Carcinoid: Rare.

Embryonal

- Rare.
- Tumors may cause **sexual precocity** or abnormal uterine bleeding.
- **β-hCG and AFP are the tumor markers** (see Table 22-2).

Mixed GCTs

- 10% of GCTs.
- Dysgerminoma and endodermal sinus tumor is the most common combination.
- **LDH, AFP,** and β-hCG may be elevated.

Treatment of Ovarian GCTs

- Surgery: **Unilateral** adnexectomy and complete surgical staging.
- Adjuvant chemotherapy: Recommended for all but stage I, grade I immature teratoma.

- Up to 80% survival with incomplete resection.
- GCTs are very chemosensitive.

BEP Therapy	Side Effects
Bleomycin	Pulmonary fibrosis
Etoposide	Blood dyscrasias
CisPlatin	Nephrotoxicity

TABLE 22-2. Ovarian Tumors and Their Serum Markers

OVARIAN TUMOR	SERUM TUMOR MARKER
Dysgerminoma	LDH
Endodermal sinus tumor	AFP
Embryonal and choriocarcinoma	β-hCG
Epithelial ovarian tumor	CA-125
GCT	Inhibin
Sertoli–Leydig cell tumor	Testosterone

Prognosis of Ovarian GCTs

Prognosis is generally good because most are discovered *early*. Five-year survival is 85% for dysgerminomas, 75% for immature teratomas, and 65% for endodermal sinus tumors.

OVARIAN SEX CORD–STROMAL TUMORS

Five to eight percent of ovarian cancers. Arise from the sex cords of the embryonic gonad before they differentiate into male or female. They are functional tumors that secrete estrogen or testosterone. They usually affect older women.

Types of Sex Cord–Stromal Tumors

Granulosa–Theca Cell Tumor

- Secretes estrogens that can cause feminization, precocious puberty, or postmenopausal bleeding.
- **Association with endometrial cancer.**
- **Inhibin is the tumor marker.**

Sertoli–Leydig Cell Tumor

- Secretes testosterone.
- Presents with **virilization, hirsutism, and menstrual disorders as a result of the testosterone.**
- **Testosterone is the tumor marker.**

Treatment of Ovarian Sex Cord–Stromal Tumors

Surgical Treatment

- **Total abdominal hysterectomy/bilateral salpingo-oophorectomy.**
- **Unilateral** oophorectomy in young women with low-stage/grade neoplasia.

Adjuvant Therapy

Data are inconclusive, but chemotherapy and radiation play a small role at present.

FALLOPIAN CELL CARCINOMA

Fallopian cell carcinomas usually are adenocarcinomas. They spread through the peritoneal fluid in a similar fashion to ovarian cancer. It is very rare and can affect any age.

Classic Presenting Triad

- Pain
- Vaginal bleeding
- Leukorrhea

Fallopian cell carcinoma is the least common gynecologic malignancy.

In any postmenopausal bleeding or discharge that cannot be explained by endometrial biopsy, fallopian cell carcinoma should be considered.

Many are diagnosed during a laparotomy for other indications.

Hydrops tubae perfluens is the pathognomonic finding, defined as cramping pain relieved with watery discharge.

Staging, Treatment, and Prognosis

All similar to ovarian cancer.

Vulvar Dysplasia and Cancer

Vulvar Intraepithelial Neoplasia (VIN)   226

Vulvar Cancer   226

Vaginal Cancer   227

VULVAR INTRAEPITHELIAL NEOPLASIA (VIN)

Dysplastic lesions of the vulva that have potential to progress to carcinoma: Etiology is unknown, although human papillomavirus (HPV) has been implicated because of similarity in pathology and often concomitant presence of cervical intraepithelial neoplasia (CIN).

Risk Factors

Risk factors for vulvar dysplasia include HPV, herpes simplex virus type II (HSV-II), lymphogranuloma venereum (LGV), pigmented moles, and poor hygiene.

Like cervical cancer, vulvar cancer risk factors include HPV types 16, 18, 31, and 33, and the precancerous lesions are classified as intraepithelial neoplasia (termed VIN as opposed to CIN).

Presentation

Pruritus and/or irritation (recent or long-standing), raised white lesions.

Diagnosis

- **Biopsy**
- Colposcopic exam (must include cervix, vagina, perineal and perianal skin)

Staging

Most common site of vulvar dysplasia is labia majora.

As in cervical dysplasia, VIN is based on degree of epithelial spread:

VIN I—involvement of < ½ epithelium

VIN II—involvement of > ½ epithelium

VIN III—full-thickness involvement (carcinoma-in-situ)

Treatment

Treatment is according to the size of the lesion:
- Small, well-circumscribed VIN: Wide local excision
- Multifocal lesions: Laser vaporization
- Extensive lesions: Vulvectomy

VULVAR CANCER

Vulvar cancer is the fourth most common gynecologic cancer (4–5% of all gynecologic cancers) and can arise as carcinoma of various types:
- Squamous (90%)
- Adenocarcinoma (Paget's disease, Bartholin's gland)
- Basal cell carcinoma
- Melanoma
- Metastasis
- Sarcoma
- Verrucous carcinoma

Most often found in women 60–70 years old.

TABLE 23-1. Staging of Vulvar Cancer

STAGE	5-YEAR SURVIVAL RATE POST TREATMENT
I: < 2-cm tumor, no spread	> 90%
II: > 2-cm tumor, no spread	> 90%
III: Spread to unilateral nodes or vagina or anus or lower urethra	Correlates to number of positive nodes: 1 node ≈ 85% ≥ 3 nodes ≈ 15%
IV: Mucosa, bilateral nodes IVa: Spread to upper urethra, rectum IVb: Distant metastases	< 10%

Signs and Symptoms

- Pruritus (most common)
- Ulceration
- Mass (often exophytic)
- Bleeding

Risk Factors

- Same as vulvar dysplasia (HPV, HSV-II, LGV, pigmented moles, and poor hygiene)
- Smoking
- Immunodeficiency syndromes

Diagnosis

Biopsy of the suspicious lesion

Staging

See Table 23-1 for staging of vulvar cancer.

Treatment

Stages I–II

Radical vulvectomy and lymphadenectomy (wide local excision is sometimes possible for certain small lesions < 1 cm).

Stages III–IV

As above, plus removal of affected organs and adjunct radiation therapy.

VAGINAL CANCER

- Vaginal cancer is a rare gynecologic malignancy (2% of gynecologic cancers).

Pruritus is the most common symptom of vulvar cancer. Always biopsy itchy white lesion on exam questions.

Clear cell adenocarcinoma of the vagina often correlates with in utero diethylstilbestrol exposure; these patients often present young.

Vulvar Dysplasia and Cancer

- Usually presents in **postmenopausal women.**
- Most common type is squamous cell carcinoma (other types are the same as vulvar cancer types).

Signs and Symptoms

- Ulcerated mass
- Exophytic mass
- Bleeding
- Asymptomatic

Diagnosis

Biopsy of suspicious lesion.

Staging

See Table 23-2 for staging of vaginal cancer.

Treatment

Stages I–II
Surgical resection and radiation

Stages III–IV
Radiation only

TABLE 23-2. **Staging of Vaginal Cancer**

STAGE	5-YEAR SURVIVAL RATE POST TREATMENT
I: Limited to vaginal mucosa	≈ 75%
II: Beyond mucosa but not involving pelvic wall	≈ 70%
III: Pelvic wall involvement	≈ 35%
IV: Involvement of bladder, rectum, or distant mets	< 15%

Gestational Trophoblastic Neoplasia

Definition   230

Hydatidiform Mole   230

Choriocarcinoma   232

Placental Site Trophoblastic Tumor (PSTT)   233

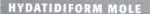
Gestational trophoblastic neoplasias (GTNs) are neoplasms arising from placental syncytiotrophoblasts and cytotrophoblasts (fetal tissue). They represent an aberrant fertilization event.

The four tumors are:
- Hydatidiform mole (complete or partial)
- Persistent/invasive trophoblastic disease
- Choriocarcinoma
- Placental site trophoblastic tumor

HYDATIDIFORM MOLE

Complete Mole

A placental (trophoblastic) tumor forms when a maternal ova devoid of deoxyribunocleic acid (DNA) is "fertilized" by the paternal sperm (see Figure 24-1):

Karyotype: Most have karyotype 46,XX, resulting from sperm penetration and subsequent DNA replication. Some have 46,XY, believed to be due to two paternal sperms simultaneously penetrating the ova.

Epidemiology: Incidence is:
- 1/1,500 pregnancies in the United States
- 1/200 in Mexico
- 1/125 in Taiwan

Partial Mole

A mole with a fetus or fetal parts (see Figure 24-2). Women with partial (incomplete) molar pregnancies tend to present later than those with complete moles:

Karyotype: Usually 69,XXY, and contains both maternal and paternal DNA.

Epidemiology: 1/50,000 pregnancies in the United States.

DNA of complete mole is always paternal.

DNA of a partial mole is both maternal and paternal.

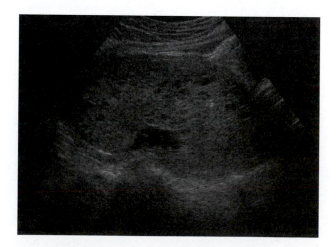

FIGURE 24-1. Complete mole on ultrasonography.

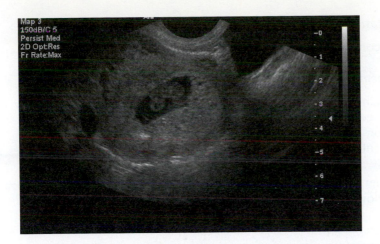

FIGURE 24-2. **Partial mole on ultrasonography.**

Invasive Mole

A hydatidiform mole that invades the myometrium: It is by definition malignant, and thus treatment involves complete metastatic workup and appropriate malignant/metastatic therapy (see below).

Histology of Hydatidiform Mole

- Trophoblastic proliferation
- Hydropic degeneration (swollen villi)
- Lack/scarcity of blood vessels

Signs and Symptoms

- Passage of vesicles (look like grapes)
- Preeclampsia < 20 weeks
- Abnormal painless bleeding in first trimester
- Uterus large for gestational age

Diagnosis

- Elevated hCG (usually > 100,000 mIU/mL)
- Absence of fetal heartbeat
- Ultrasound—"snowstorm" pattern
- Pathologic specimen—grapelike vesicles
- Histologic specimen (see above)

Treatment of Complete or Partial Moles

- Dilation and curettage (D&C) to evacuate and terminate pregnancy.
- Follow-up with the workup to rule out invasive mole (malignancy):
  - Chest x-ray (CXR) to look for lung mets.
  - Liver function tests to look for liver mets.
  - hCG monitoring: Weekly until normal for 3 weeks, then monthly until normal for 6 months; yearly for 1–3 years. If the hCG level rises, does not fall, or falls and then rises again, the molar pregnancy is considered persistent/malignant.
  - Contraception should be used during the 1-year follow-up.

A young woman who passes grape-like vesicles from her vagina should be diagnosed with hydatidiform mole.

All early (< 20 weeks) preeclampsia is molar pregnancy until **proven** otherwise.

GTNs secrete human chorionic gonadotropin (hCG), lactogen, and thyrotropin.

Ten to 15% of complete moles will be malignant. Two percent of partial moles will be malignant.

Metastatic Workup

CXR, computed tomography (CT) of brain, lung, liver, kidneys.

Treatment (for Nonmetastatic Molar Pregnancies)

- Chemotherapy—methotrexate or Actinomycin D (as many cycles as needed until hCG levels return to normal)
  or
- Total abdominal hysterectomy + chemotherapy (fewer cycles needed)

Treatment for metastatic molar pregnancy is the same as for choriocarcinoma (see below).

Any of the following on exam indicates molar pregnancy:
- Passage of grapelike vesicles
- Preeclampsia early in pregnancy
- Snowstorm pattern on ultrasound

CHORIOCARCINOMA

An epithelial tumor that occurs with or following a pregnancy (including ectopic pregnancies, molar pregnancies, or abortion):

Histopathology: Choriocarcinoma has characteristic sheets of trophoblasts with extensive hemorrhage and necrosis, and unlike the hydatidiform mole, choriocarcinoma has no villi.

Epidemiology: Incidence is about 1/16,000 pregnancies.

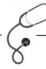

Nonmetastatic malignancy has almost a 100% remission rate following chemotherapy.

Diagnosis

- Increased hCG
- Absence of fetal heartbeat
- Uterine size/date discrepancy
- Specimen (sheets of trophoblasts, no villi)

Sheets of trophoblasts = choriocarcinoma.

As with invasive mole and malignant hydatidiform mole, a full metastatic workup is required when choriocarcinoma is diagnosed.

Treatment of Nonmetastatic Choriocarcinoma and Prognosis

- Chemotherapy—methotrexate or Actinomycin D (as many cycles as needed until hCG levels return to normal)
  or
- Total abdominal hysterectomy + chemotherapy (fewer cycles needed)

Remission rate is near 100%.

Treatment of Metastatic Choriocarcinoma, Metastatic Invasive Mole, or Metastatic Hydatidiform Mole

Treatment is determined by the patient's risk (high or low) or prognostic score.

Prognostic Group Clinical Classification

Low risk:
- hCG < 100,000 IU/24-hr urine or < 40,000 mIU/mL serum.
- < 4 months from antecedent pregnancy event or onset of symptoms to treatment.
- No brain or liver metastasis.
- No prior chemotherapy.
- Pregnancy event is not a term pregnancy.

High risk: Opposite of above (i.e., hCG > 100,000 IU/24-hr urine, > 4 months from pregnancy, brain or liver mets, etc.).

PSTT is a rare form of GTN. It is characterized by infiltration of the myometrium by intermediate trophoblasts, which stain positive for human placental lactogen. Unlike other GTN, hCG is only slightly elevated.

Treatment

Total abdominal hysterectomy: Prognosis is poor if there is tumor recurrence or metastasis.

World Health Organization (WHO) Prognostic Scoring System

	SCORE			
RISK FACTOR	0	1	2	4
Age (years)	≤ 39	> 39		
Pregnancy	H. mole	Abortion	Term	
Interval from pregnancy event to treatment (in months)	< 4	4–6	7–12	> 12
hCG (IU/mL)	< 10^3	10^3–10^4	10^4–10^5	> 10^5
ABO blood group (female × male)		O × A A × O	B AB	
Number of metastases		1–4	5–8	> 8
Site of metastasis		Spleen Kidney	GI Liver	Brain
Size of largest tumor (cm)		3–5	> 5	
Prior chemotherapy agent		Single	Multiple	

Scores are added to give the prognostic score.

Treatment According to Score/Prognostic Factors

Low risk (score ≤ 4)	Single-agent therapy (methotrexate)	Remission rate 90 to 99%
Intermediate risk (score 5 to 7)	Multiple-agent therapy (MAC therapy—methotrexate, actinomycin, and cyclophosphamide)	Remission rate ≈ 50%
High risk (score ≥ 8)	Multiple-agent therapy (EMACO therapy—etoposide, MAC, and vincristine)	

Sexually Transmitted Diseases and Vaginitis

Pelvic Inflammatory Disease (PID)	236
Gonorrhea	237
Chlamydia	238
Syphilis	238
Genital Herpes	239
Human Immunodeficiency Virus (HIV) and Acquired Immune Deficiency Syndrome (AIDS)	240
Human Papillomavirus (HPV)	240
Chancroid	241
Pediculosis Pubis (Crabs)	241
Vaginitis	242
Toxic Shock Syndrome	243

Definition

Inflammation of the female upper genital tract (uterus, tubes, ovaries, ligaments) caused by ascending infection from the vagina and cervix.

Common Causative Organisms

- *Neisseria gonorrhoeae*
- *Chlamydia trachomatis*
- *Escherichia coli, Peptostreptococcus*
- *Gardnerella vaginalis*

Diagnosis

Physical Exam

- Abdominal tenderness
- Adnexal tenderness
- Cervical motion tenderness

Rarely is a single organism responsible for PID, but always think of chlamydia and gonorrhea first.

Lab Results and Other Possible Exam Signs

- +/– Fever
- Gram-positive staining
- Pelvic abscess
- Elevated white count, erythrocyte sedimentation rate (ESR), C-reactive protein (CRP)
- Purulent cervical discharge
- Culture evidence of *N. gonorrhoeae* or *C. trachomatis*

Laparoscopy

This is the "gold standard" for diagnosis, but it is usually employed only in cases unresponsive to medical treatment.

Requirement for diagnosis of PID:
1. Abdominal tenderness
2. Adnexal tenderness
3. Cervical motion tenderness
Positive lab tests are not necessary for diagnosis.

Risk Factors

- Age < 35 years
- Multiple sexual partners
- New sex partner(s)
- Unprotected intercourse
- Concomitant history of sexually transmitted disease
- Presence of intrauterine contraceptive device

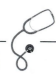

Chandelier sign—when you touch the cervix, there is so much pain that she jumps to the chandelier.

Criteria for Hospitalization

- Pregnancy, adolescence (as they can have an unpredictable course)
- Peritonitis
- Gastrointestinal (GI) symptoms (nausea, vomiting)
- Abscess (tubo-ovarian or pelvic)
- Uncertain diagnosis
- Surgical emergency
- Outpatient failure or intolerance
- Lack of compliance
- Pelvic abscess
- Immunocompromised

HIGH-YIELD FACTS

Sexually Transmitted Diseases

Treatment

Inpatient
Cefoxitin/cefotetan + doxycycline (preferred for chlamydia)
Clindamycin + gentamicin (preferred for abscess)

Outpatient
Ceftriaxone + doxycycline or tetracycline. Alternatively, if patient does not tolerate doxycycline/tetracycline, substitute with erythromycin.

Sexual partners should also be treated empirically.

Criteria for hospitalization
for PID:
GU PAP
GI symptoms
Uncertain diagnosis

Peritonitis
Abscess
Pregnancy

GONORRHEA

An infection of the urethra, cervix, pharynx, or anal canal, caused by the gram-negative diplococcus, *Neisseria gonorrhoeae*.

There is a 50–90% chance of transmission after one exposure to gonorrhea.

Presentation

- Asymptomatic
- **Dysuria**
- **Endocervicitis**
- **Vaginal discharge**
- PID

Diagnosis

- Culture in Thayer–Martin agar (gold standard)
- Gonazyme (enzyme immunoassay)
- DNA probe
- DNA/polymerase chain reaction (PCR) amplification

Fifteen percent of women with gonorrhea will progress to PID if untreated.

Treatment

Ceftriaxone 125 mg IM single dose
or
Cefixime 400 mg PO single dose
or
Ciprofloxacin 500 mg PO single dose
or
Ofloxacin 400 mg PO single dose

If coinfection with chlamydia is not ruled out:
Azithromycin 2 g PO single dose
or
Doxycycline 100 mg PO bid × 7 days

Sexual partners should also be treated.

When treating gonorrhea, empirical treatment of chlamydial coinfection is also given.

Chlamydia is twice as common as gonorrhea.

Fitz-Hugh–Curtis perihepatitis presents as right upper quadrant pain, fever, nausea, and vomiting. It can be caused by gonorrhea or chlamydia.
- ↑ Liver function tests
- "Violin string" adhesions

Use erythromycin rather than doxycycline for pregnant women or children with chlamydia.

Physicians often treat both gonorrhea and chlamydia even if diagnosing only one.

CHLAMYDIA

Chlamydia is an infection of the genitourinary (GU) tract, GI tract, conjunctiva, nasopharynx, caused by *Chlamydia trachomatis*, an obligate intracellular bacteria.

Presentation

There are numerous serotypes of chlamydia generally speaking. Serotypes A–K cause more localized GU manifestations and the L serotypes a systemic disease (lymphogranuloma venereum).

Serotypes A–K

Serotypes A–K of *Chlamydia trachomatis* can have the following presentation:
- Asymptomatic
- **Mucopurulent discharge**
- **Cervicitis**
- **Urethritis**
- PID
- Trachoma—conjunctivitis resulting in eyelash hypercurvature and eventual blindness from corneal abrasions
- Fitz-Hugh–Curtis syndrome
- Reiter syndrome if accompanied by arthritis and inflammation of the eye and urethra

Serotypes L1–L3

Serotypes L1–L3 of *Chlamydia trachomatis* cause **lymphogranuloma venereum.** This is a systemic disease that can present in several forms:
- Primary lesion: Painless papule on genitals
- Secondary stage: Lymphadenitis
- Tertiary stage: Rectovaginal fistulas, rectal strictures

Diagnosis

- Microimmunofluorescence test (MIF)—measures antichlamydia immunoglobulin M (IgM) titers. Titer > 1:64 is diagnostic.
- Isolation in tissue culture.
- Enzyme immunoassay.
- Nucleic acid amplification.
- DNA probe.

Treatment

Doxycyline 100 mg bid × 7 days or azithromycin 2 g PO single dose/erythromycin.

SYPHILIS

Syphilis is an infection caused by the spirochete *Treponema pallidum*.

Presentation

Syphilis has various stages of manifestation that present in different ways:

Sexually Transmitted Diseases

HIGH-YIELD FACTS

- Primary syphilis: **Painless hard chancre** of the vulva, vagina, or cervix (or even anus, tongue, or fingers), usually appearing 1 month after exposure: Spontaneous healing after 1–2 months.
- Secondary syphilis: **Generalized rash** (often palms and soles), condyloma lata, mucous patches with lymphadenopathy, fever, malaise, usually **appearing 1 to 6 months after primary chancre**: Spontaneous regression after about 1 month.
- Tertiary syphilis (latent stage): **Presents years later** with skin lesions, bone lesions (gummas), cardiovascular lesions (e.g., aortic aneurysms), central nervous system (CNS) lesions (e.g., tabes dorsalis).

Diagnosis

- Screening is done via rapid plasma reagin (RPR) or Venereal Disease Research Laboratory (VRDL). These are nonspecific and can give positive results for many conditions.
- Treponemal test (FTA-ABS) is a very specific test, performed if RPR is positive.
- Visualization of spirochetes on darkfield microscopy is an additional test available.

Treatment

- **Benzathine penicillin G** for all stages, though in differing doses.
- Doxycycline, if penicillin allergic.

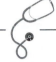

Pregnancy may give false-positive RPR.

GENITAL HERPES

- Infection caused by herpes simplex virus type I (HSV-I) in 85% of cases, and by HSV-II in 15% of cases.
- HSV is a DNA virus.
- Fifteen percent of adults have antibodies to HSV-II, most without history of infection.

Presentation

Patients with herpes can be asymptomatic, in addition to the following:
- **Primary infection: Painful multiple vulvar vesicles,** *associated with fever, lymphadenopathy, malaise,* usually 1 to 3 weeks after exposure.
- **Recurrent infection:** Recurrence from viral stores in the sacral ganglia, resulting in a *milder version* of primary infection including vesicles.
- **Nonprimary first episode:** This is defined as **initial infection by HSV-II** in the presence of *preexisting antibodies to HSV-I* or vice versa. The preexisting antibodies to HSV-II can make the presentation of HSV-I milder.

Major Risks

- Cervical cancer
- Neonatal infection

Diagnosis

- Gross examination of vulva for typical lesions
- Cytologic smear—multinucleated giant cells (Tzanck test)
- Viral cultures

Stress, illness, and immune deficiency are some factors that predispose to herpes recurrence.

Treatment

Treatment for HSV is palliative and not curative.

- *Primary outbreak*—acyclovir 400 mg tid × 7 days.
- *Recurrent infection*—one half original dose of acyclovir.
- *Pregnancy*—acyclovir during third trimester.
- A vaccine is under development.
- Famciclovir and valacyclovir are newer antivirals that are dosed less frequently.

HUMAN IMMUNODEFICIENCY VIRUS (HIV) AND ACQUIRED IMMUNE DEFICIENCY SYNDROME (AIDS)

HIV is an RNA retrovirus and causes AIDS. The virus infects CD4 lymphocytes and other cells and causes decreased cellular immunity.

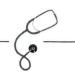

Presentation

- **Initial infection:** Mononucleosis-like illness occurring weeks to months after exposure—fatigue, weight loss, lymphadenopathy, night sweats. This is followed by a long asymptomatic period lasting months to years.
- **AIDS:** Opportunistic infections, dementia, depression, Kaposi's sarcoma, wasting.

Risk Factors

- Intravenous drug use
- Blood transfusions between 1978 and 1985
- Prostitution
- Multiple sex partners/unprotected sex
- Bisexual or homosexual partners

Diagnosis

- **Enzyme-linked immunosorbent assay (ELISA):** Detects antibodies to HIV. It is sensitive but not as specific.
- **Western blot:** Done for confirmation if ELISA is positive. It is very specific.
- **PCR:** An alternative means of testing.

Treatment

Two antiretroviral agents plus one protease inhibitor has been common treatment.

HUMAN PAPILLOMAVIRUS (HPV)

HPV causes genital warts (**condylomata acuminata**):
- Subtypes 6 and 11 are not associated with cervical or penile cancer.
- Subtypes 16, 18, 31, and 33 are associated with cervical and penile cancer.

Presentation

Warts of various sizes (sometimes described as cauliflower-like) on the external genitalia, anus, cervix, or perineum.

Diagnosis

- Warts are diagnosed by visualization.
- Cervical dysplasia caused by HPV infection is screened via Pap smear.

Treatment

- Condylomata acuminata are treated with cryosurgery, laser ablation, or trichloroacetic acid.
- See Cervical Dysplasia chapter for treatment of cervical dysplasia.

CHANCROID

Presentation

Chancroid presents as a papule on external genitalia that becomes a painful ulcer (unlike syphilis, which is painless) with a gray base. Inguinal lymphadenopathy also is possible.

Etiology

Haemophilus ducreyi.

Diagnosis

Gram stain of ulcer or inguinal node aspirate showing gram-negative rods.

Treatment

Ceftriaxone, erythromycin, or azithromycin.

PEDICULOSIS PUBIS (CRABS)

Presentation

Pruritus in the genital area from parasitic saliva.

Etiology

Blood-sucking parasite *(Phthirus pubis).*

Diagnosis

Visualization of crabs or nits, history of pruritus.

Treatment

Pyrethrin cream or Lindane shampoo.

Lactobacillus, the normal flora in the vagina, creates an acidic environment that kills most other bacteria. Raising the pH allows other bacteria to survive.

Definition

Vaginitis is inflammation of the vagina, often resulting in increased discharge and/or pruritus, and usually caused by an identifiable microbe (see Table 25-1).

Etiology

- **Antibiotics**: Destabilize the normal balance of flora
- **Douche**: Raises the pH
- **Intercourse**: Raises the pH
- **Foreign body**: Serves as a focus of infection and/or inflammation

TABLE 25-1. Vaginitis

	PHYSIOLOGIC (NORMAL)	BACTERIAL VAGINOSIS	CANDIDIASIS	TRICHOMONIASIS
Clinical complaints	None	**Malodorous discharge,** especially after menses, intercourse	**Pruritus, erythema, edema,** odorless discharge, dyspareunia	**Copious, frothy discharge,** malodorous, pruritus, urethritis
Quality of discharge	Clear or white, no odor	Homogenous **gray** or white, **thin,** sticky	White, **"cottage cheese–like"**	Green to **yellow,** sticky, **"bubbly"** or "frothy"
pH	3.8–4.2	**> 4.5**	4–4.5	**> 4.5**
Microscopic findings	Epithelial cells Normal bacteria include mostly *Lactobacillus,* with *Staphylococcus epidermidis, Streptococcus,* as well as small amounts of colonic flora	Visualize with saline **Clue cells** (epithelial cells with bacteria attached to their surface) Bacteria include *Gardnerella (Haemophilus)* and/or *Mycoplasma*	**In 10% KOH Budding yeast** and pseudohyphae	In saline Motile, **flagellated, protozoa**
"Whiff" test	Negative (no smell)	**Positive** (fishy smell)	Negative	Positive or negative
Treatment		Oral or topical **metronidazole** or topical **clindamycin**	Oral, topical, or suppository **imidazole** (or other various antifungals)	Oral **metronidazole** (*Note:* Metronidazole has potential disulfiram-like reaction and has a metallic taste)
Treat sexual partners?		Not necessary	Not necessary	**Yes**

There are several common organisms that cause vaginitis: Bacterial (*Gardnerella*), *Candida*, and *Trichomonas*. The distinguishing features are described with the following characteristics.

Diagnostic Characteristics

- **Clinical characteristics.**
- **Quality of discharge.**
- **pH**—secretions applied to test strip reveal pH of discharge.
- **"Whiff" test**—combining vaginal secretions with 10% KOH: Amines released will give a fishy odor, indicating a positive test.
- **Microscopic findings.**

TOXIC SHOCK SYNDROME

See Figure 25-1.

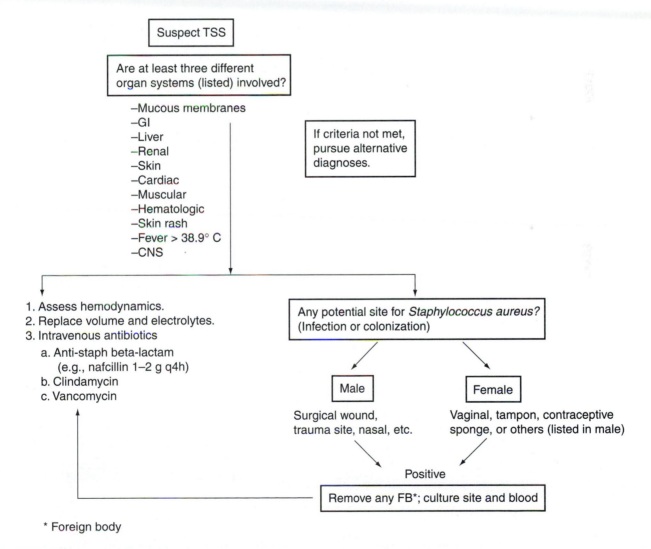

FIGURE 25-1. Toxic shock syndrome (TSS) workup.

(Modified, with permission, from Pearlman MD, Tintinalli JE, eds. *Emergency Care of the Woman.* New York: McGraw-Hill, 1998: 615.)

Vulvar Disorders

Vulvar Dystrophies 246

Psoriasis 246

Vestibulitis 246

Cysts 247

VULVAR DYSTROPHIES

Vulvar dystrophies are a group of disorders characterized by various pruritic, white lesions of the vulva. Lesions must be biopsied to rule out malignancy.

Lichen Simplex Chronicus (LSC)

LSC is a hypertrophic dystrophy caused by chronic irritation resulting in the raised, whitened appearance of hyperkeratosis. Lesions may also appear red and irritated due to itching. Microscopic examination reveals acanthosis and hyperkeratosis.

Lichen Sclerosis

An atrophic lesion characterized by paperlike appearance on both sides of the vulva and epidermal contracture leading to loss of vulvar architecture: Microscopic examination reveals epithelial thinning with a layer of homogenization below and inflammatory cells.

Lichen Planus

White, inflamed or erosive lesions that are painful. May lead to synechiae. May present as vulvo-vaginal-gingival syndrome.

Treatment of Vulvar Dystrophies

- Steroid cream (hydrocortisone)
- Diphenhydramine at night to prevent itching during sleep

Lichen simplex chronicus and lichen sclerosis carry no increased risk of malignancy.

PSORIASIS

Psoriasis is a common dermatologic condition that is characterized by red plaques covered by silver scales. Although it commonly occurs over the knees and/or elbows, lesions can be found on the vulva as well. Pruritus is variable.

Treatment

- Steroid cream
- Coal tar with ultraviolet light therapy or topical vitamin D

VESTIBULITIS

Inflammation of the vestibular glands that leads to tenderness, erythema, and pain associated with coitus (insertional dypareunia and/or postcoital pain): Etiology is unknown. Although the affected area turns white with acetic acid under colposcopic examination, these lesions are not dysplastic.

Treatment

- Temporary sexual abstinence.
- Trichloroacetic acid.
- Xylocaine jelly for anesthesia.
- Surgery—if lesions are unresponsive to treatment, vestibulectomy is possible, though with risk of recurrence.

CYSTS

Bartholin's Abscess

Bartholin's abscesses occur when the main duct draining Bartholin's gland is occluded, which usually occurs due to infection. Inflammatory symptoms generally arise from infection and can be treated with antibiotics.

Treatment

- Incision and drainage and marsupialization (suturing the edges of the incised cyst to prevent reocclusion)

  or

- Ward catheter (a catheter with an inflatable tip left in the gland for 10 to 14 days to aid healing)

Sebaceous Cysts

Sebaceous cysts occur beneath the labia majora (rarely minora) when sebaceous gland ducts are occluded. Besides the palpable, smooth mass, patients are generally asymptomatic. Infection or other complications can be treated with incision and drainage.

Hidradenomas

Hidradenomas (apocrine sweat gland cysts) also occur beneath the labia majora as a result of ductal occlusion. These cysts tend to be more pruritic than sebaceous cysts. They are also treated by incision.

Other Rare Cysts

Cyst of canal of Nuck: A hydrocele (persistent processus vaginalis), contains peritoneal fluid

Skene's duct cyst: Ductal occlusion and cystic formation of the Skene's (paraurethral) glands

The vestibular glands (Bartholin's glands) are located at the 5 and 7 o'clock positions of the inferolateral vestibule (area between the labia minora).

Bartholin's glands are analogous to the male Cowper's gland (bulbourethral gland). It secretes a thick alkaline fluid during coitus.

Vulvar Disorders

HIGH-YIELD FACTS

Vulvar Disorders

Menopause

Definitions	250
Factors Affecting Age of Onset	250
Physiology During the Perimenopausal Period	250
Physiology During the Menopausal Period	251
Treatment of the Adverse Effects of Menopause	251

Average age of menopause in the United States is about 51 years.

Cigarette smoking is the only factor shown to significantly reduce age of menopause (3 years).

FSH levels double to ≈ 20 mIU/mL in perimenopause and triple to ≈ 30 in menopause.

DEFINITIONS

- **Menopause** is the *final menstruation* marking the termination of menses (defined as 6–12 months of amenorrhea).
- Menopause is preceded by the **climacteric** or **perimenopausal period**, the multiyear transition from optimal menstrual condition to menopause.
- The **postmenopausal period** is the time after menopause.
- See Figure 27-1.

FACTORS AFFECTING AGE OF ONSET

- Genetics
- Smoking (decreases age by 3 years)
- Chemo/radiation therapy

PHYSIOLOGY DURING THE PERIMENOPAUSAL PERIOD

Oocytes Die

- Women's immature eggs, or **oocytes, begin to die** precipitously (apoptosis) and become **resistant to follicle-stimulating hormone (FSH)**, the pituitary hormone that causes their maturation.
- **FSH levels rise** for two reasons:

1. Decreased inhibin (inhibin inhibits FSH secretion; it is produced in smaller amounts by the fewer oocytes).
2. Resistant oocytes require more FSH to successfully mature, triggering greater FSH release.

Stages:	-5	-4	-3	-2	-1	0	+1	+2
Terminology:	Reproductive			Menopausal Transition			Postmenopause	
	Early	Peak	Late	Early	Late*		Early*	Late
				Perimenopause				
Duration of Stage:	variable			variable		(a) 1 yr	(b) 4 yrs	until demise
Menstrual Cycles:	variable to regular	regular		variable cycle length (>7 days different from normal)	≥2 skipped cycles and an interval of amenorrhea (≥60 days)	Amen x 12 mos	none	
Endocrine:	normal FSH		↑ FSH	↑ FSH			↑ FSH	

*Stages most likely to be characterized by vasomotor symptoms   ↑ = elevated

Final Menstrual Period (FMP)

FIGURE 27-1. The STRAW staging system.

(Reproduced, with permission, from Soules MR et al. Executive Summar: Stages of Reproductive Aging Workshop (STRAW). *Fertil Steril* 2001;76(5):874–878.)

Ovulation Becomes Less Frequent

Women **ovulate less frequently,** initially one to two fewer times per year and, eventually, just before menopause, perhaps once every 3–4 months. This is due to a **shortened follicular phase.** The luteal phase does not change.

Estrogen Levels Fall

Estrogen (estradiol-17β) **levels begin to decline,** resulting in **hot flashes** (may also be due to increased luteinizing hormone [LH]). Hot flashes usually occur on the face, neck, and upper chest and last a few minutes, followed by intense diaphoresis.

Oligo/anovulation leads to abnormal bleeding in perimenopause.

PHYSIOLOGY DURING THE MENOPAUSAL PERIOD

- **Decrease in estradiol level.**
- **FSH and LH levels rise** secondary to absence of negative feedback.
- Androstenedione is aromatized peripherally to estrone (less potent than estradiol). Major estrogen in postmenopausal women.
- Androstenedione and testosterone levels fall.

The most **important physiologic change** that occurs with menopause is the **decline of estradiol-17β** levels that occurs with the cessation of follicular maturation. Table 27-1 lists the organ systems affected by those decreased estradiol levels.

When menopause occurs after age 55, it is considered late menopause.

TREATMENT OF THE ADVERSE EFFECTS OF MENOPAUSE

Hormone replacement therapy (HRT) or estrogen replacement therapy (ERT) has been shown to counteract some of the complications of estradiol loss listed in Table 27-1.

Estrogen Replacement Therapy

ERT = estrogen only: Indicated in women status post hysterectomy.

Hormone Replacement Therapy

HRT = estrogen + progesterone: The progesterone component is needed to protect the endometrium from constant stimulation and resultant increase in endometrial cancer. It is indicated for women who still have their uterus.

The Women's Health Initiative and the Heart and Estrogen/Progestin Replacement Study (HERS) have prompted great changes in the understanding and remediations of HRT.

- Cardiovascular: HRT does not seem to protect against cardiovascular disease. In fact, it could make it worse.

TABLE 27-1. **Physiologic Effects of Menopause and HRT**

Organ System	Effect of Decreased Estradiol	Available Treatment
Cardiovascular	↑ LDL, ↓ HDL After two decades of menopause, the risk of myocardial infarction (MI) and coronary artery disease is equal to that in men.	
Bone	Osteoporosis. Estrogen receptors found on many cells mediating trabecular bone maintenance (i.e., ↑ osteoblast activity, ↓ osteoclast activity).	▪ HRT/ERT becoming second line ▪ Calcitonin ▪ Raloxifene ▪ Etidronate (a bisphosphonate osteoclast inhibitor) ▪ Exercise ▪ Calcium supplementation 50% reduction in death from hip fracture with normal estrogen levels
Vaginal mucous membranes	Dryness and atrophy, with resulting dyspareunia, atrophic vaginitis.	▪ HRT/ERT pill or cream
Genitourinary	Loss of urethral tone, dysuria.	▪ HRT/ERT
Psychiatric	Lability, depression.	▪ +/− HRT/ERT, antidepressants
Neurologic	Preliminary studies indicate there may be a link between low levels of estradiol and Alzheimer's disease.	▪ HRT/ERT
Hair and skin	Skin—less elastic, more wrinkled. Hair—male growth patterns.	▪ HRT/ERT pill or cream

ERT = estrogen replacement therapy; HDL, high-density lipoprotein; HRT, hormone replacement therapy; LDL, low-density lipoprotein.

Although HRT recommendations changed with the WHI study, there are many flaws in the design. Recommendations will likely change in the near future.

- Osteoporosis: Controversial because they protect against osteoporosis but there are other medications such as bisphosphonates and raloxifene that can do the same thing.
- Breast cancer: Seen to increase the risk of breast cancer.

Recommendations

- Short-term therapy (< 5 years) is acceptable for menopausal symptom relief.
- Osteoporosis can be prevented with HRT; however, other medications are as effective and could be used as first-line therapy.
- HRT should not be used to prevent cardiovascular disease.

Risks of HRT/ERT

- Increase risk of breast cancer
- Increase incidence in endometrial cancer (ERT only)
- Thromboembolism
- Cholecystitis/cholelithiasis

Contraindications to HRT/ERT

- Unexplained vaginal bleeding
- Breast carcinoma (relative, not absolute, contraindication)
- Metastatic endometrial carcinoma/ovarian carcinoma
- Liver disease
- History of thromboembolic disease
- History of MI

Estrogen creates a hypercoagulable state due to increased production of hepatic coagulation factors.

Menopause

Pelvic Relaxation

Anatomy of Pelvic Floor Support   256

Prolapse   256

Urinary Incontinence   259

Several crucial structures make up the support of the female pelvic floor. Disturbance of any of the following can result in prolapse:

- Bony structure
- Broad and round ligaments
- Endopelvic fascia
- Pelvic diaphragm
- Urogenital diaphragm
- Perineum

The pelvic diaphragm is made up of the levator ani and coccygeal muscles.

PROLAPSE

Prolapse is the downward displacement of an organ from its normal position. There are several types.

Types

Prolapses can be classified according to the location of the protruding structure: Anterior, apical, and posterior.

Anterior
- Cystocele (bladder)—see Figure 28-1
- Cystourethrocele

Apical
- Uterocele
- Vaginal prolapse

Posterior
- Rectocele—see Figure 28-1
- Enterocele (intestine)—see Figure 28-1

In general, think of prolapse as either limited to the upper vagina, to the introitus, or protruding from the body.

Grading

Organ displacement:

■ To the level of the ischial spines	Grade I
■ Between ischial spines and introitus	Grade II
■ Within introitus	Grade III
■ Past introitus	Grade IV

Risk Factors

Many conditions can cause prolapse by disturbing the anatomical supports (childbirth), disrupting the innervations, or increasing the pressure load. The following are some examples:

- Increased load: Obesity, cough (e.g., chronic obstructive pulmonary disease)
- Loss of levator ani function: Postpartum
- Disturbance of parts: Postsurgical

Anything that increases pelvic pressure can cause a prolapse:
- Constipation
- Chronic obstructive pulmonary disease
- Tumor/mass

HIGH-YIELD FACTS

Pelvic Relaxation

256

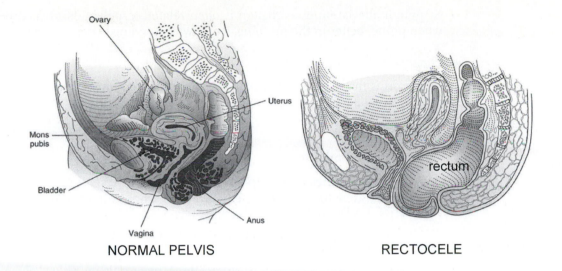

NORMAL PELVIS   RECTOCELE

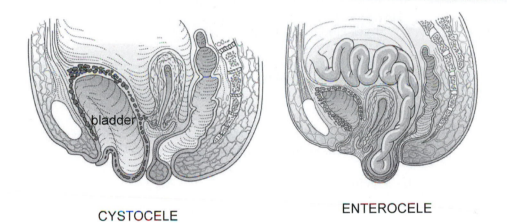

CYSTOCELE   ENTEROCELE

FIGURE 28-1. **Types of prolapse.**

(Reproduced, with permission, from Pernoll ML. *Benson & Pernoll's Handbook of Obstetrics and Gynecology*, 10th ed. New York: McGraw-Hill, 2001: 807–808.)

- Loss of innervation: Amyotrophic lateral sclerosis (ALS), paralysis
- Loss of connective tissue: Spina bifida, myelomeningocele

Signs and Symptoms

- Feeling of "pressure"
- Organ protrusion, especially upon exertion
- Incontinence
- Groin pain
- Dyspareunia
- Spotting

Symptom alleviation/exacerbation is often related to pelvic effort (i.e., better when prone, better in the morning, worse with standing, worse in evening).

Diagnosis

Diagnosis is made by direct visualization of prolapsed organ during complete pelvic examination: Patient should be examined in the standing position.

Treatment

Asymptomatic Prolapse

- Usually requires **follow-up** but no immediate intervention.
- Pelvic-strengthening exercises (i.e., **Kegel** maneuvers) and/or HRT/ERT may benefit.

Symptomatic Prolapse

Can be treated with a pessary or surgically. A **pessary** is an object placed in the upper vagina designed to help maintain support of the pelvic organs. Types include:

    Smith-Hodge (oval ring)
    Doughnut (ring)
    Inflatable
    Gehrung (U-shaped)

Surgical Treatment

These are several types of surgical repairs for each type of prolapse. New, minimally invasive techniques are being developed.

Cystocele

- **Anterior colporrhaphy:** Bladder buttress base sutures proximal to the bladder neck.
- **Kelly plication** (anterior vaginal repair): Endopelvic fascial reinforcement via vaginal approach.
- **Lefort procedure**/colpocleisis: Surgical obliteration of the vaginal canal.
- **Burch/Marshall–Marchetti–Krantz** procedures: Urethrovescicular suspension via abdominal approach.
- **Sling procedure**: Elevation of bladder neck and urethra via vaginal and abdominal approaches.

Rectocele

Posterior repair: Posterior vaginal wall reinforcement with levator ani muscles via vaginal approach.

Enterocele

Moschovitz repair: Approximation of endopelvic fascia and uterosacral ligaments via abdominal approach to prevent an enterocele. Similar transvaginal repair exists.

Uterine Prolapse

Hysterectomy: A uterine prolapse often occurs in conjunction with another prolapse, and so combined repairs are usually performed.

Definition

Involuntary loss of urine that is a symptom of a pathological condition. Incontinence can be due to reversible or irreversible (but treatable) causes.

Reversible Causes

Delerium, infection, atrophic vaginitis, drug side effects, psychiatric illness, excessive urine production, restricted patient mobility, and stool impaction are *reversible* causes of urinary incontinence.

It is helpful to search out these easily correctable causes before moving on to the more expensive and invasive workup for the irreversible causes.

Irreversible Types

Stress Incontinence

Loss of urine (usually **small amount**) only *upon increased intra-abdominal pressure* (i.e., with coughing, laughing, exercise): Caused by **urethral hypermotility** and/or **sphincter dysfunction** that maintains enough closing pressure at rest but not with exertion.

Urge Incontinence

Sudden feeling of **urgency** followed by **complete emptying** of bladder: Caused by **unopposed detrusor contraction.**

Overflow Incontinence

Constant **dribbling** +/− urgency with **inability to completely empty the bladder:** Caused by **detrusor underactivity** (due to a neuropathy) or **urethral obstruction.**

Mixed Incontinence

Combinations of above.

Evaluation

History

Ask about aforementioned symptoms, medications, medical history (diabetes mellitus, neuropathies).

Physical

- Pelvic exam: Check for cystoceles, urethroceles, and atrophic changes.
- Rectal exam: Check for impaction and rectocele; assess sphincter tone.
- Neuro exam: Assess for neuropathy.

Labs

Urinalysis and culture to rule out urinary tract infection.

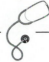

Reversible causes of urinary incontinence: **"DIAPPERS"**
Delerium
Infection
Atrophic vaginitis
Pharmacologic causes
Psychiatric causes
Excessive urine production
Restricted mobility
Stool impaction

Total incontinence = continuous urinary and/or fecal leakage due to previous pelvic surgery, obstetric trauma, radiation, or fistula formation.

Remember to examine for prolapse while patient is standing.

Q-tip test: Increased upward motion of the Q-tip is caused by loss of support from the urethrovesicular junction, indicating stress incontinence.

Q-Tip Test

A cotton swab is placed in the urethra. The change in angle between the Q-tip and the woman's body is measured upon straining. Normal upward change is < 30 degrees, and a **positive test** is one with **> 30-degree change. A positive test indicates stress incontinence.**

Cystometry

Cystometry provides measurements of the **relationship of pressure and volume in the bladder.** Catheters that measure pressures are placed in the bladder and rectum, while a second catheter in the bladder supplies water to cause bladder filling. Measurements include residual *volume, pressures at which desires to void occur, bladder compliance, flow rates,* and *capacity.* Diagnoses: Stress, urge, and overflow incontinence.

Urodynamic Studies

A set of studies that evaluate lower urinary tract function. Studies may include **cystometry** (see above), **bladder filling tests, cystoscopy, uroflowmetry leak-point pressure tests,** to name a few. Can help diagnose all types of incontinence.

Treatment

STRESS INCONTINENCE

- **Kegel exercises** strengthen urethral muscles.
- **Estrogen therapy.**
- **α-adrenergic drugs.**
- Surgical repair (usually Burch procedure or Kelly plication).

URGE INCONTINENCE

- **Medications:**
  - Anticholinergics
  - Calcium channel blockers
  - Tricyclics
- **Timed voiding:** Patient is advised to urinate in prescribed hourly intervals before the bladder fills.
- Surgery is rarely used to treat urge incontinence.
- Avoid stimulants and diuretics (i.e., alcoholic beverages, coffee, carbonated beverages).

OVERFLOW INCONTINENCE

Due to Obstruction
Relieve obstruction.

Due to Detrusor Underactivity
Treat possible neuro causes:
- **Diabetes mellitus**
- B_{12} deficiency

TOTAL INCONTINENCE

Surgical repair for fistulas.

Women's Health

Health Maintenance and Screening Tools 262

Preventive Health Information 264

Substance Abuse 265

Seat Belt Use 265

Safer Sex Practices 266

Female Sexual Response and Sexual Expression 266

Disorders of Sexual Dysfunction 267

Domestic Violence 270

Sexual Assault 271

Ethics 272

Office Health Maintenance Tests 274

This chapter focuses on women's health, ages 13 through the postmenopausal years.

Pap Smear

- Yearly 3 years after initiation of sexual activity but no later than age 21.
- After three consecutive normal Paps in a healthy, low-risk female, screening may be done every 2–3 years.

Manual Breast Exams

- An annual breast exam should be performed on all women beginning at age 13.
- *All women, especially by age 30, should perform self-breast exams once per month (e.g., premenopausal women should examine their breasts one week after their menstrual period).*

Mammography

- Annually beginning at age 35 if there is family history of breast cancer or 10 years prior to family member diagnosis
- Annually beginning at age 40 for all others

Colon Cancer Screening

- Fecal occult blood testing beginning at age 40–50 years
- Sigmoidoscopy starting at age 50, every 5 years (if higher risk, start earlier)
  or
- Colonoscopy every 10 years (especially if inflammatory bowel disease, colonic polyps, colon cancer, or a family history of familial polyposis coli, colorectal cancer, or cancer family syndrome)

Laboratory Testing

THYROID-STIMULATING HORMONE (TSH)

Test:
- At age 65 and older, check every 3–5 years
- Periodic screening (age 19–64) if strong family history of thyroid disease and if autoimmune disease

CHOLESTEROL

Test:
- Every 5 years beginning at age 20
- Every 3–5 years between ages 65 and 75
Periodic screening if:
- Familial lipid disorder
- Family history of premature coronary artery disease (CAD) (< 55 years)
- History of CAD

LIPIDS

Periodic screening if:
- Elevated cholesterol
- History of parent or sibling with blood cholesterol ≥ 240 mg/dL
- History of sibling, parent, or grandparent with premature (< 55 years) CAD
- Diabetes mellitus (DM)
- Smoker
- Obese

FASTING GLUCOSE

Test:
- Every 3 years beginning at age 45
- Every 3–5 years if:
  - Family history of DM (one first- or two second-degree relatives)
  - Obese
  - History of gestational DM
  - Hypertension
  - High-risk ethnic group

Tuberculosis (TB) Skin Testing

Recommended for:
- Regular testing for teens.
- Human immunodeficiency virus: HIV-positive people should be tested regularly.
- Exposure to TB-infected person requires testing.
- Medically underserved/low-income populations.

Sexually Transmissible Infection Testing

Recommended for:
- History of multiple sexual partners
- History of sex with a partner who has multiple sexual contacts
- Persons whose partner has a sexually transmitted disease (STD)
- History of STD

HIV Testing

Recommended for women:
- Seeking treatment for STDs
- With a history of prostitution/intravenous drug abuse
- With a history of sex with an HIV-positive partner
- Whose partners are bisexual
- Who were transfused between 1978 and 1985
- In an area of high prevalence of HIV infection
- With recurrent genital tract disease
- < 50 years of age who have invasive cervical cancer
- Who are pregnant or planning to become pregnant

Routine screening for chlamydial and gonorrheal infection is recommended for all sexually active adolescents and high-risk females, even if they are asymptomatic.

Bacteriuria Testing/Urinalysis

- Periodically for women with DM and women ≥ 65 years of age
- During routine prenatal care

Immunizations

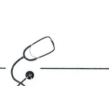

See Table 5-2 for immunizations during pregnancy.

- Tetanus–diphtheria booster once between 13 and 16 years
- Tetanus–diphtheria booster every 10 years
- Measles, mumps, rubella (MMR) for all nonimmune women
- Hepatitis B vaccine for those not previously immunized
- Varicella vaccine if not immune
- Hepatitis A vaccine if at high risk
- Influenza vaccine annually beginning at age 55
- Give influenza vaccine prior to age 55 if:
  - Residents of chronic care facilities
  - Immunosuppression
  - Hemoglobinopathies
  - **Women who will be in T2 or T3 during the endemic season**
- Pneumococcal vaccine if 65 years of age, or sooner for women with:
  - Sickle cell disease
  - Asplenia
  - Alcoholism/cirrhosis
  - Influenza vaccine risk factors

PREVENTIVE HEALTH INFORMATION

Nutrition and Exercise

The issues of nutrition and body weight should be emphasized during the three major transitional periods in a woman's life:

1. Puberty
2. Pregnancy
3. Menopause

One's body weight is determined by three major factors:

1. Genetics and heredity, which control:
   - Resting metabolic rate
   - Appetite
   - Satiety
   - Body fat distribution
   - Predisposition to physical activity
2. Nutrition
3. Physical activity and exercise

GOALS

1. Maintain a healthy diet consisting of frequent small meals (i.e., four to six instead of two to three):
   - Utilize the Food Guide Pyramid as a tool in making food choices in daily life.

High-fat diets have adverse effects on lipid metabolism, insulin sensitivity, and body composition, even in the absence of weight gain.

- Adjust caloric intake for age and physical activity level:
    - As one ages, there is a decrease in resting metabolic rate and loss of lean tissue.
    - Older women who are physically active are less likely to lose lean tissue and can maintain their weight with higher caloric intake.
2. Physical activity during all stages of life should include exercise at moderate intensity for 30 minutes on most days of the week.

Exercise will increase the body's metabolic rate and prevent the storage of fat.

SUBSTANCE ABUSE

Alcohol

Women experience more accelerated and profound medical consequences of excessive alcohol than men (a phenomenon called "telescoping"):

- Cirrhosis
- Peptic ulcers that require surgery
- Myopathy
- Cardiomyopathy
- When combined with cigarette smoking, leads to oral and esophageal cancers
- Fetal alcohol syndrome:
    - Teratogenic effects are dose related.
    - Includes growth retardation, facial anomalies, mental retardation.

Alcohol:
- Accounts for 100,000 deaths per year in the United States.
- Excessive use for women is about one half the quantity considered excessive for men.
- When compared to men, women have relatively reduced activity of gastric alcohol dehydrogenase to begin alcohol metabolism and have less body water in which to distribute unmetabolized alcohol.

Cigarettes

- Linked to lung cancer and coronary artery disease (CAD).
- Most common factor in chronic obstructive pulmonary disease.
- **Endocrine effects:** Smokers reach menopause earlier and have increased risk of osteoporosis.
- **Obstetric effects:** Reduced fertility, increased rates of spontaneous abortion, premature delivery, low-birth-weight infants, reduced head circumferences, abruption.
- Children who grow up exposed to secondhand smoke have higher rates of respiratory and middle ear illness.

- Lung cancer is the most common cause of cancer death in women.
- Related to 400,000 deaths per year.

SEAT BELT USE

- Deaths due to accidents are greatest in women aged 13–39.
- Accidents cause more deaths than infectious diseases, pulmonary diseases, diabetes, and liver and kidney disease.
- Motor vehicle accidents account for 50,000 deaths per year and > 4–5 million injuries per year.
- Seat belts decrease chance of death and serious injury by > 50%.

HIGH-YIELD FACTS

Women's Health

SAFER SEX PRACTICES

Improved and successful prevention of pregnancy and STDs by more adolescents requires counseling that includes:

- Encouragement to postpone sexual involvement
- Provision of information about contraceptive options, including emergency contraception and side effects of various contraceptive methods

FEMALE SEXUAL RESPONSE AND SEXUAL EXPRESSION

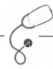

Adolescent pregnancy and abortion rates in the United States are higher than in any other developed country.

Female Response Cycle

Consists of:

Desire
- Begins in the brain with perception of erotogenic stimuli via the special senses or through fantasy.

Arousal
- Clitoris becomes erect.
- Labia minora become engorged.
- Blood flow in the vaginal vault triples.
- Upper two thirds of the vagina dilate.
- Lubricant is secreted from the vaginal surface.
- Lower one third of vagina thickens and dilates.

After somatosensory stimulation, orgasm is an adrenergic response.

Plateau
- The formation of transudate (lubrication) in the vagina continues in conjunction with genital congestion.
- Occurs prior to orgasm.

Orgasm
- Rhythmic, involuntary, vaginal smooth muscle and pelvic contractions, leading to pleasurable cortical sensory phenomenon ("orgasm").

Unlike men, women have no refractory period and can experience multiple orgasms without a time lag in between.

Sexuality: Resolution (Prenatal Through Childhood)

Resolution
- Sexual development begins prenatally when the fetus differentiates into a male or female.
- Sexual behavior, usually in the form of masturbation, is common in childhood.
- As children grow older, they are socialized into cultural emphases on privacy and sexual inhibition in social situations.
- Between ages 7 and 8, most children engage in childhood sexual games, either same-gender or cross-gender play.

It is normal for children < 6 years of age to be curious about their own or others' bodies, and they may engage in observable sexual behaviors.

Adolescence

Gender identity and sexual preferences begin to solidify as puberty begins.

Menstrual Cycle

The menstrual cycle can affect sexuality (i.e., in some women, there is a peak in sexual activity in the midfollicular [postmenstrual] phase).

Pregnancy

For some women, intercourse is avoided during pregnancy due to fear of harming the baby or a self-perception of unattractiveness. Coitus is safe until 36 weeks in normal pregnancies.

Sexual intercourse during pregnancy is NOT related to bacterial vaginosis or preterm birth in normal, healthy pregnancies. But there are certain obstetrical conditions in which coitus should be avoided (i.e., placenta previa, abruptio placentae, premature labor, and premature rupture of membranes).

Postpartum

- Women often experience sexual problems within the first 6 months of delivery.
- Problems may include:
    - Perineal soreness
    - Excessive fatigue
    - Disinterest in sex

Menopause

- A decrease in sexual activity is most frequently observed.
- Advancing age is associated with decreased:
    - Intercourse frequency.
    - Orgasmic frequency.
    - Enjoyment of sexual activity: Sexual enjoyment may also be decreased with the increased duration of the relationship and with the partner's increasing age.
- Decreased sexual responsiveness may be reversible if caused by reduction in functioning of genital smooth muscle tissue.
- Psychosocially, middle-aged women often feel less sexually desirable.

Little is known about how being a new mother affects sexual desire and response.

Hormonal Changes

- Estrogen decrease leads to decreased vaginal lubrication, thinner and less elastic vaginal lining.
- Estrogen decrease leads to depressive symptoms, resulting in decreased sexual desire and well-being.

DISORDERS OF SEXUAL DYSFUNCTION

It is important to first clarify whether the dysfunction reported is:
- *Lifelong or acquired?*
- *Global* (across all partners) *or situational?*

General Evaluation Strategies

Differentiate between the following possible etiologies:
- Medical illnesses
- Menopausal status
- Medication use (antihypertensives, cardiovascular meds, antidepressants, etc.)

Rule out other psychiatric/psychological causes:
- Life content (stress, fatigue, relationship problems, traumatic sexual history, guilt)
- Major depression
- Drug abuse
- Anxiety
- Obsessive–compulsive disorder

General Management Strategies

- Medical illnesses need evaluation and specific treatment.
- Screen for and treat depression with psychotherapy or medication.
- Reduce dosages or change medications that may alter sexual interest (i.e., switch to antidepressant formulations that have less of an impact on sexual functioning such as bupropion [Wellbutrin] or nefazodone [Serzone]).
  or
- Combine buspirone (Buspar), an antianxiety agent, with a selective serotonin reuptake inhibitor to counteract the sexual side effects.
- Address menopause and hormonal deficiencies.

Sexual Desire Disorders

- **Hypoactive sexual desire disorder**—persistent or recurrent absence or deficit of sexual fantasies and desire for sexual activity.
- **Sexual aversion disorder**—persistent or recurrent aversion to and avoidance of genital contact with a sexual partner.

Sexual Arousal Disorder

- Partial or total lack of physical response as indicated by lack of lubrication and vasocongestion of genitals.
- Persistent lack of subjective sense of sexual excitement and pleasure during sex.

Management

- Treat decreased lubrication with KY Jelly or Astroglide.
- Menopausal symptoms may respond to oral or topical estrogen.
- Sildenafil (Viagra) may be helpful.
- Refer for psychosocial consultation or therapy if psychological issues exist.

Orgasmic Disorder

Persistent delay or absence of orgasm.

Evaluation

Differentiate between the following:
- Take sexual experience into account—women often become more orgasmic with experience.
- Physical factors that may interfere with neurovascular pelvic dysfunction (i.e., surgeries, illnesses, or injuries).

Complaints of sexual arousal disorder are typically accompanied by complaints of dyspareunia, lack of lubrication, or orgasmic difficulty.

Lack of orgasm during intercourse is considered a normal variation of female sexual response if the woman is able to experience orgasm with a partner using other, noncoital methods.

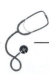

Sildenafil citrate (Viagra) and other vasodilators are currently undergoing clinical trials with women for sexual dysfunction treatment.

- Psychological and interpersonal factors are very common (i.e., growing up with messages that sex is shameful and for men's pleasure only).
- Partner's lack of sexual skills.

Management

For lifelong, generalized orgasmic disorder, there is rarely a physical cause. Treat with masturbation programs and/or sex therapy.

Sexual Pain Disorders

DYSPAREUNIA

Recurrent genital pain before, during, or after intercourse.

Evaluation

Differentiate between:
- Physical disorder
- Vaginismus
- Lack of lubrication

Management

- If due to vaginal scarring/stenosis due to history of episiotomy or vaginal surgery, vaginal stretching with dilators and massage.
- If postmenopausal, vaginal estrogen cream to improve vaginal pliability.
- Low-dose tricyclic antidepressants may be helpful.
- Pelvic floor physical therapy (Kegel exercises).
- Coital position changes.

VAGINISMUS

Recurrent involuntary spasm of the outer third of the vagina (perineal and levator ani muscles) interfering with or preventing coitus.

Evaluation

- Obtain history.
- Rule out organic causes (i.e., vaginitis, endometriosis, pelvic inflammatory disease, irritable bowel syndrome, urethral syndrome, interstitial cystitis, etc.).
- Examine the pelvis for involuntary spasm.
- Rule out physical disorder or other psychiatric disorder.

Management

- Treat organic causes.
- Psychotherapy.
- Provide reassurance.
- Physical therapy (i.e., Kegel exercises, muscle relaxation massage, and gradual vaginal dilatation) (the woman controls the pace and duration).

Exogenous administration of estrogen improves vaginal lubrication, atrophic conditions, hot flashes, headaches, and insomnia.

Menopause and sexual dysfunction: Menopause → vaginal atrophy and lack of adequate lubrication → painful intercourse → decreased sexual desire.

Many antidepressants alter sexual response by increasing the availability of serotonin and decreasing dopamine.

Estrogen improves overall sense of well-being—probably secondarily improves sexual desire.

HIGH-YIELD FACTS

Women's Health

Domestic violence refers to a relationship in which an individual is victimized (physically, psychologically, or emotionally) by a current or past intimate partner.

Recognition of the Occurrence of Domestic Violence

- Injuries to the head, eyes, neck, torso, breasts, abdomen, and/or genitals.
- Bilateral or multiple injuries.
- A delay between the time of injury and the time at which treatment is sought.
- Inconsistencies between the patient's explanation of the injuries and the physician's clinical findings.
- A history of repeated trauma.
- The perpetrator may exhibit signs of control over the the health care team, refusal to leave the patient's side to allow private conversation, and control of victim.
- The patient calls or visits frequently for general somatic complaints.
- **In pregnant women:** Late entry into prenatal care, missed appointments, and multiple repeated complaints are often seen in abused pregnant women.

Assessment

See Table 29-1.

Reaction to Domestic Violence

- Listen in a nonjudgmental fashion, and assure the patient that it is not her fault, nor does she deserve the abuse.

TABLE 29-1. Abuse Assessment Screen

1. Have you ever been emotionally or physically abused by your partner or someone important to you?
2. Within the last year, have you been hit, slapped, kicked, or otherwise physically hurt by someone?
3. Since you've been pregnant, have you been hit, slapped, kicked, or otherwise physically hurt by someone?
4. Within the last year, has anyone forced you to have sexual activities? Has anyone in the past forced you to have sexual activities?
5. Are you afraid of your partner or anyone you listed above?

Source: Nursing Research Consortium on Violence and Abuse, 1989. Reproduced, with permission, from Seltzer VL, Pearse WH. *Women's Primary Health Care,* 2nd ed. New York: McGraw-Hill, 2001: 659.

- Assess the safety of the patient and her children.
- If the patient is ready to leave the abusive relationship, connect her with resources such as shelters, police, public agencies, and counselors.
- If the patient is not ready to leave, discuss a safety or exit plan and provide the patient with domestic violence information.
- Carefully document all subjective and objective findings. The records can be used in a legal case to establish abuse.

In general, where the performance of one duty conflicts with the other, the preferences of the patient prevail.

SEXUAL ASSAULT

Sexual assault occurs when any sexual act is performed by one person on another without that person's consent.

Rape is defined as sexual intercourse without the consent of one party, whether from force, threat of force, or incapacity to consent due to physical or mental condition.

Sexual abuse occurs in approximately two thirds of relationships involving physical abuse.

Rape-Related Post-Traumatic Stress Disorder (RR-PTSD)

A "rape-trauma" syndrome resulting from the psychological and emotional stress of being raped.

Signs and Symptoms

Acute Phase
- Eating and sleep disorders
- Vaginal itch, pain, and discharge
- Generalized physical complaints and pains (i.e., chest pain, backaches, and pelvic pain)
- Anxiety/depression

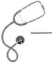

Any injury during pregnancy, especially one to the abdomen or breasts, is suspicious for abuse.

Reorganization Phase
- Phobias
- Flashbacks
- Nightmares
- Gynecologic complaints

Management

Physician's Medical Responsibilities
- Obtain complete medical and gynecologic history.
- Assess and treat physical injuries in the presence of a female chaperone (even if the health care provider is female).
- Obtain appropriate cultures.
- Counsel patient and provide STD prophylaxis.
- Provide preventive therapy for unwanted pregnancy.
- Assess psychological and emotional status.
- Provide crisis intervention.
- Arrange for follow-up medical care and psychological counseling.

Because abuse may begin later in pregnancy or after the baby is born, pregnant women should be questioned about abuse during each trimester and postpartum.

Physicians are not obligated to perform procedures if they are morally opposed to them or give advice on sexual matters that they are ignorant of, but should refer patients as necessary.

The greatest risk of danger of spousal abuse is around a threat or attempt to leave the relationship.

The annual incidence of sexual assault is 73 per 100,000 females.

Seventy-five percent of rape victims know their perpetrator.

Physician's Legal Responsibilities

- Obtain informed consent for treatment, collection of evidence, taking of photographs, and reporting of the incident to the authorities.
- Accurately record events.
- Accurately describe injuries.
- Collect appropriate samples and clothing.
- Label photographs, clothing, and specimens with the patient's name; seal and store safely.

Treatment

Infection Prophylaxis

- Gonorrhea, chlamydia, and trichomonal infections:
  - Ceftriaxone 125 mg IM + azithromycin 1 g PO in a single dose
  or
  - Doxycycline 100 mg PO bid for 7 days + metronidazole 2 g PO in a single dose
- Offer the hepatitis B vaccine.
- Administer tetanus–diphtheria toxoid when indicated.

Postcoital Regimen

- **Combined estrogen–progestin pills:** Ovral (50 ug ethinyl estradiol, 0.5 mg norgestrel): 2 tabs PO STAT, then 2 more tabs 12 hours later:
  - 75% effective
- **Mifepristone (RU 486):** A single dose of 600 mg PO:
  - 99.9% effective

ETHICS

It is the physician's responsibility to:
- Determine the patient's preferences.
- Honor the patient's wishes when the patient can no longer speak for herself.

End-of-Life Decisions

- **Advanced directives (living will and durable power of attorney for health care)** allow patients to voice their preferences regarding treatment if faced with a potentially terminal illness.
- In a **living will,** a competent, adult patient may, in advance, formulate and provide a valid consent to the withholding/withdrawal of life-support systems in the event that injury or illness renders that individual incompetent to make such a decision.
- In a **durable power of attorney for health care,** a patient appoints someone to act as a surrogate decision maker when the patient cannot participate in the consent process.

Life-Sustaining Treatment

Any treatment that serves to prolong life without reversing the underlying medical condition.

Reproductive Issues

The ethical responsibility of the physician is:
- To identify his or her own opinions on the issue at hand.
- To be honest and fair to their patients when they seek advice or services in this area.
- To explain his or her personal views to the patient and how those views may influence the service or advice being provided.

Informed Consent

A legal document that requires a physician to obtain consent for treatment rendered, an operation performed, or many diagnostic procedures.

Informed consent requires the following conditions be met:

1. Must be **voluntary**
2. **Information:**
   - **Risks and benefits** of the procedure are discussed.
   - **Alternatives** to procedure are discussed.
   - **Consequences** of not undergoing the procedure are discussed.
   - Physician must be willing to **discuss the procedure** and answer any questions the patient has.
3. The patient must be **competent.**

Exceptions

The following are certain cases in which informed consent need not be obtained:

1. Lifesaving medical emergency.
2. Suicide prevention.
3. Normally, minors must have consent obtained from their parents. However, minors may give their own consent for certain treatments, such as alcohol detox and treatment for venereal diseases.

Patient Confidentiality

The information disclosed to a physician during his or her relationship with the patient is confidential. The physician should not reveal information or communications without the express consent of the patient, unless required to do so by law.

Exceptions

- A patient threatens to inflict serious bodily harm to herself or another person.
- Communicable diseases.
- Gunshot wounds.
- Knife wounds.

Minors

When minors request confidential services, physicians should encourage minors to involve their parents.

Where the law does not require otherwise, the physician should permit a competent minor to consent to medical care and should *not* notify the parents without the patient's consent.

If the physician feels that without parental involvement and guidance the minor will face a serious health threat, and there is reason to believe that the parents will be helpful, disclosing the problem to the parents is equally justified.

OFFICE HEALTH MAINTENANCE TESTS

STARTING AGE	TEST	HOW OFTEN?
13–16	■ Tetanus–diphtheria booster	Once
> 16	■ Tetanus–diphtheria booster	Every 10 years
≥ 18 *(or before if sexually active)*	■ Pap smear	Annually
	■ Manual breast exams	
	■ CBC, BUN, creatinine, hemoglobin	Periodically
≥ 20	■ Cholesterol	Every 5 years
≥ 40	■ Mammogram	Annually
	■ Fecal occult blood testing	
≥ 45	■ Fasting glucose	Every 3 years
≥ 50	■ Sigmoidoscopy	■ Every 5 years
	or	
	■ Colonoscopy if high risk	■ Every 10 years
≥ 55	■ Influenza vaccine	Annually
≥ 65	■ TSH	Every 3–5 years
	■ Cholesterol	
	■ Urinalysis	Periodically
	■ Pneumococcal vaccine	Once

BUN, blood urea nitrogen; CBC, complete blood count; TSH, thyroid-stimulating hormone.

Awards for Obstetrics and Gynecology

▶ Awards and Opportunities

▶ Web Sites of Interest

Emory University Program in Family Planning and Human Sexuality

Ten-week internship offering research and providing educational and clinical experiences in the field of reproductive health. $1,500 stipend. March 1 deadline.

MARCH OF DIMES SUMMER SCIENCE RESEARCH

A program designed for medical students willing to spend 3 months working in a laboratory or clinical setting devoted primarily to research in birth defects. The first step is for the Dean's office to submit to the March of Dimes one or two names of individuals on the staff who are actively engaged in birth defects research. These staff people will be requested by the March of Dimes to provide the names of two students each. Although a maximum of four names will be provided, only two can be selected from each school. Stipend is $1,000 per student. Deadline: January 15.

March of Dimes Research Support on Reproductive Hazards in the Workplace

A program designed to recognize and ultimately detect adverse reproductive effects in occupationally exposed women and men. Deadline: February 1.

National Osteoporosis Foundation Student Fellowship

Eight-week to 4-month fellowship for research related to the causes and prevention of osteoporosis. The research may be either clinical or basic under the supervision of an established investigator. Maximum award $4,000. Deadline: March 31.

AMWA STUDENT LOAN FUND

This fund with lenient payback terms continues to provide AMWA member medical students with financial help when they are most in need. With the escalating costs of a medical school education, AMWA's loans provide students with much-needed financial assistance when they face huge resource needs. Women who are enrolled in accredited U.S. medical or osteopathic medicine schools, who are U.S. citizens or permanent residents and who are student members of national AMWA are eligible to apply for a loan. For an application or additional information, contact Marie Glanz, at (703) 838-0500 or e-mail mglanz@amwa-doc. org.

AMWA WILHELM-FRANKOWSKI SCHOLARSHIP

This scholarship was offered for the first time in 1996 and was made possible through the generous bequests of Drs. Hazel Wilhelm and Clementine Frankowski. The $4,000 medical student scholarship, awarded for community service, activity in women's health issues, and participation in AMWA and other women-in-medicine groups, is now awarded annually to an AMWA student member. Medical students attending an accredited U.S. medical or osteopathic medicine school in their first, second, or third year are eligible to apply. Applications are mailed from January through mid-April of each year. Contact AMWA at <amwa-doc.org> for additional information and to be placed on the mailing list to receive a scholarship application. Deadline for receipt of completed applications is April 30. Supporting documentation deadline is May 15.

COUNTRY DOCTOR SCHOLARSHIP PROGRAM

$10,000 annually, $40,000 aggregate

Georgia residents qualify for funding to obtain primary care medical degrees such as IM, General Surgery, OB/GYN, Peds, and FP. In return, the student must practice in a Georgia board-approved town of 15,000 or less population. APPLICATION DEADLINE: May 15. Contact: Joe B. Lawley, PhD, State Medical Education Board, 270 Washington St SW, 7th Floor, Room 7093, Atlanta, GA 30334.

AWHS OVERSEAS ASSISTANCE GRANT

The American Women's Hospitals Service provides assistance with transportation costs (airfare, train fare, etc.—up to $1,500) connected with pursuing medical studies in an off-campus setting where the medically neglected will benefit.

Grants are awarded to national AMWA members completing their second, third, or fourth year at an accredited U.S. medical or osteopathic medicine school or a resident who will be spending a minimum of six weeks and no longer than one year in a sponsored program, which will serve the needs of the medically underserved.

The program must be sponsored by your school, another school, or an outside agency or, if there is no sponsor, it must be a program for which your school takes responsibility and provides academic credit.

Contact Marie Glanz at (703) 838-0500 or mglanz@amwa-doc. org to obtain further details about this opportunity and request an application.

BPW CAREER ADVANCEMENT SCHOLARSHIP FOR WOMEN

$500 to $1,000 grants for women over 25 in their third or fourth year of studies with critical need for assistance. APPLICATION DEADLINE: April 15. Contact: Scholarships/Loans Business and Professional Woman's Foundation, 2012 Mass Ave NW, Washington, DC 20036. Tel: (202) 293-1200 ext. 169.

Alpha Omega Alpha Research Fellowships

The purpose of the fellowships is to stimulate interest in re-search among medical students. Areas of research may include clinical investigation, basic research, epidemiology, and the social sciences, as related to medicine. The program is designed to stimulate students who have not had prior research experience. Fellowship is for $2,000. Deadline: January.

AMA-MSS Councils

The Medical student section of the AMA (AMA-MSS) has several councils for which it seeks medical students.

Application involves a current curriculum vitae, an essay on why you want to be a member of an AMA Council, which Council(s) you prefer, what you consider to be your major strengths and qualifications for the position, and what benefits you feel are likely to result from your participation.

- Council on Constitution and Bylaws
- Council on Ethical and Judicial Affairs
- Council on Legislation
- Council on Long Range Planning and Development
- Council on Medical Education
- Council on Medical Service
- Council on Scientific Affairs

AMA-MSS Committee Application

Medical students are sought to serve on the following AMA-MSS committees:

- Committee on Computers and Technology (formerly Computer Projects Committee)
- Committee on Long Range Planning
- Legislative Affairs Committee
- Minority Issues Committee
- Ad Hoc Committee on Community Service and Advocacy
- Ad Hoc Committee on Membership Recruitment and Retention
- Ad Hoc Committee on MSS Programs and Activities
- Ad Hoc Committee on Scientific Issues Committee (CSI)
- Ad Hoc Committee on International Health and Policy

All applications must be completed and submitted with a CV to American Medical Association, Department of Medical Student Services, 515 North State Street, Chicago, IL 60610. Fax: (312) 464-5845.

AMA POLITICAL ACTION COMMITTEE (AMPAC)

AMPAC is a bipartisan group that serves to advance the interest of medicine within Congress, specifically by supporting candidates for office that are friendly to medicine. They also provide numerous programs to educate physicians, medical students, and their families on political activism. The Board directs the programs and activities of this extremely important political action committee. Adding medical students to the leadership of this group will provide for better medical student representation within the group, as well as greater student involvement in this important process. Terms are for two years.

Editorial Positions with Medical Student JAMA

MS/JAMA is the seven- to eight-page medical student section of the Journal of the American Medical Association (JAMA) that appears in the first JAMA of every month, September through May, and is also produced each month on the MS/JAMA Web site. As a regular section of a major medical journal, produced by and for medical students, MS/JAMA represents a unique opportunity to train to become journal editors, writers, and contributors. The MS/JAMA Web site is located at www.ama-assn.org/ms-jama.

AMA Foundation Leadership Award Program

This award is an exciting opportunity to advance your leadership skills within organized medicine. Medical students who have demonstrated strong nonclinical leadership skills in medicine or community affairs and have an interest in further developing these skills within organized medicine are eligible. The objective of the award program is to encourage involvement in organized medicine and continue leadership development among the country's brightest and most energetic medical students and residents. Twenty-five medical students will be selected. Travel expenses for award winners, including airfare and three nights' hotel accommodation, will be paid for directly by the AMA Foundation to attend the 2001 AMA National Leadership Development Conference. For applications call (800) AMA-3211, ext. 4751 or 4746.

GOVERNMENT RELATIONS INTERNSHIP PROGRAM APPLICATION

The Department of Medical Student Services, in conjunction with the Washington office of the American Medical Association, is pleased to offer assistance to students seeking to increase their involvement and education in national health policy and in the national legislative activities of organized medicine.

Through the Government Relations Internship Program, stipends of $2,500 are available to assist selected students who are completing health policy internships in the Washington, DC, area. To be eligible for the program, students must be AMA members who have secured a policy internship in the Washington, DC, area. Through the program, students may also apply for an internship at the AMA's Washington office (two positions available) or at the Health Care Financing Administration in Baltimore, Maryland (one position available). Students participating in the program generally arrange their internships with Congressional offices, specialty societies, or federal agencies in the DC area. A list of possible internship contacts is available.

WEB SITES OF INTEREST

ACOG.org

ACOG.org is the official Web site for the American College of Obstetrics and Gynecology. The Web site has several items of interest to medical students, including a career guide for medical students interested in the specialty.

Medical student membership in ACOG

A one-time $10 fee includes:
- ACOG publications
- Reduced meeting fees
- Entry into their member-only Web site
- Updates in the specialty

<www.som.tulane.edu/student/t_3hints/OBGYN.HTM>

Some nice tips from Tulane medical school on how to impress during your OB/GYN rotation.

JOIN AMWA (American Medical Women's Association)

For a one-time fee of $52, you can become a medical student life member of AMWA. Membership benefits include:
- Networking opportunities at the national and local levels— 60 physicians branches and 120 student branches
- Continuing Medical Education (CME) programs
- Leadership and mentoring opportunities

- Professional and personal development programs
- AMWA's legislative network
- AMWA's Annual, Interim, and Regional Meetings offering career and personal development curricula
- Gender Equity Information Line to assist you with concerns on sexual harassment, gender bias, racial discrimination, and other matters
- Women's Health Advocacy
- Subscription to the *Journal of the American Medical Women's Association* (JAMWA), a quarterly peer-reviewed scientific publication
- AMWA Connections, a bimonthly newsletter keeping you connected to your colleagues
- Women's health projects and innovative "Train-the-Trainer" programs
- Discounts for AMWA publications such as *The Women's Complete Healthbook*, *The Women's Complete Wellness Book*, and *Developing a Child Care Program*
- Advanced access and reduced fees to AMWA's Career Development Institute
- Members-Only sections on the AMWA Web site

www.ncrw.org

National Council for Research on Women—An alliance of women's research and policy centers providing research, policy analysis, advocacy, and innovative programming on women and girls.

ms4c.org

Medical Students for Choice (MSFC) is dedicated to ensuring that women receive comprehensive reproductive health care, including abortion. One of the greatest obstacles to safe, legal abortion is the absence of trained providers. The more than 6,000 medical students and residents of <ms4c.org> are committed to ensuring that medical practitioners are prepared to provide their patients with the full range of reproductive health care choices.

www.ama-assn.org

- FREIDA Online—computer access to graduate training program data (members receive up to 30 free mailing labels)
- Airline discounts for travel to residency interviews (graduating seniors only)

- USP Drug Information for the Health Care Professional (free 1998 benefit for three and four multiyear membership options)
- Discounts up to 35% in AMA's Medical Student Catalog
- PaperChase—discounted online subscription to MEDLINE searches (free access after 5 P.M.)
- Policy Promotion Grants for chapter and community projects
- Educational loans consolidation thru Mellon Bank (888) 867-2116

medscape.com

This site's medical student section includes features such as "today's headlines," a medical student discussion forum to vent and exchange study tips, a weekly "focus" story from a med student's perspective, free tools for your palm pilot, test-taking skills, study tips, and a "clerkshop clues" section that summarizes the latest advances relevant to OB/GYN, Medicine, Surgery, and other clerkships.

Index

A

Abdominal exam, during pregnancy, 46
Abortion
  complete, 139, 141
  elective (induced), 141
  incomplete, 138–139, 141
  induced, 141, 147–149
  inevitable, 138, 141
  missed, 139, 141
  recurrent, 140, 141
  septic, 139–140, 141
  spontaneous, 136–137, 141
    chromosomal abnormalities and, 136
    endocrine abnormalities and, 137
    environmental factors and, 137
    immunologic factors and, 137
    infectious agents and, 136
    uterine abnormalities and, 137
  therapeutic (induced), 141
  threatened, 138
Abruptio placentae (placental abruption), 127–128
Acidemia, 75
Acidosis, 75
Acquired immune deficiency syndrome (AIDS), 240
ACTH. *See* Adrenocorticotropic hormone
Adenomyosis, 184, 187–190, 192
  vs. endometriosis, 190
Adrenal gland, 32
Adrenocorticotropic hormone (ACTH), 40
AFP. *See* Alpha-fetoprotein, 40
Albumin blood levels, during pregnancy, 26
Alcohol use in pregnancy, 98

Alpha-fetoprotein (AFP), 40
  maternal serum, 46
Amenorrhea, 172–173
Amniocentesis, 49
Amniotic fluid index (AFI), 49, 74–75
Amino acids, during pregnancy, 27
Ampulla, 17
Analgesics, use in pregnancy, 103–104
Anatomy, normal, 13–17
  cervix, 15
    blood supply, 15
    cervical epithelium, 15
    components, 15
    nerve supply, 15
  fallopian (uterine) tubes, 17
    blood supply, 17
    nerve supply, 17
    parts, 17
  ovaries, 17
    blood supply, 17
    histology, 17
    nerve supply, 17
  pelvic viscera, ligaments of, 16–17
  uterus, 15–16
    blood supply, 16
    components, 15
    histology, 16
    nerve supply, 16
  vagina, 15
    blood supply, 15
    nerve supply, 15
  vulva, 14
    blood supply, 14
    lymph, 14
    nerve supply, 14
Androgen excess, 175–178
Anemia, during pregnancy, 110
Antiasthmatics, use in pregnancy, 104

Antibiotics and anti-infective agents, use in pregnancy, 104
Anticoagulants, use in pregnancy, 102
Appendicitis, during pregnancy, 109
Apt test, 125
Artificial insemination of donor sperm, 166
Asherman syndrome, 173
Asphyxia, 75
Awards for obstetrics and gynecology, 275–279

B

Backache, during pregnancy, 54
Bacteriuria, asymptomatic, during pregnancy, 29
Bartholin's abscess, 247
Basal body temperature, 165
β-hCG, 21–22
  plasma, 22
  urine, 21
Bethesda staging system, 200
Bishop score, 62, 63
Blastocyst, 36
Bleeding
  first-trimester, 136
  third-trimester , 125–130
    circumvallate placenta, 130
    extrusion of cervical mucus ("bloody show"), 130
    fetal vessel rupture, 129–30
    placenta previa, 128–129
    placental abruption (abruptio placentae), 127–128
    uterine rupture, 130
  postcoital, 182
  postmenopausal, 181–182
  premenopausal, abnormal, 180–181
  uterine, abnormal, 179–182

Blood, postpartum changes in, 90
Blood pressure, during pregnancy, 25
"Bloody show," 60, 130
Body mass index (BMI), 51
Braxton Hicks contractions (false labor), 59
Breast-feeding, 94–95
  benefits, 94
  contraindications to, 94–95
  recommended dietary allowances, 94
Breast–ovarian cancer syndrome, 219
Breasts
  mammography, 262
  manual exams, 262
  postpartum changes in, 89
    colostrum, 90
      mature milk and lactation, 90
      milk, development of, 89
      milk-secreting machinery, development of, 89
Breech presentations, 66, 67
Broad ligament, 16

C

CA-125, 192, 218
Caffeine, in pregnancy, 52
Cardiac output, during pregnancy, 28
Cardinal ligament, 17
Cardiovascular drugs, use in pregnancy, 104
Cardiovascular disease, and pregnancy, 107–108
  Eisenmenger syndrome, 108
  mitral stenosis, 107–108
  mitral valve prolapse, 108
Cardiovascular system, during pregnancy, 28–29
Central nervous system, during pregnancy, 28
Central venous pressure, during pregnancy, 25
Cervical canal, 15
Cervical cancer, 198, 203–210
  clear cell adenocarcinoma of, 210
  differential diagnosis, 204
  epidemiology, 204
  grading of, 208
  recurrent, 208–210
  risk factors for, 198

staging of invasive, 206
symptoms, 204
TNM category staging, 207
treatment for bulky central pelvic disease, 208
treatment of invasive, 205
types of, 204–205
  adenocarcinoma, 205
  metastases, sites of, 205
  metastatic to cervix by direct extension, 205
  squamous cell, 204–205
Cervical cap, 154–155
Cervical dysplasia, 197–202
  colposcopy with cervical biopsy and endocervical curettage, 201
  cone biopsy and LEEP, 201–202
  cryotherapy, 202
  laser therapy, 202
  overview, 198
  Pap smear, 198–200
  risk factors for, 198
  squamocolumnar junction (SCJ), 198
Cervical exam, during labor, 62
Cervical ripening, 35
Cervix, 15
  antibacterial mucous plug of, 35
  blood supply, 15
  cervical epithelium, 15
  components, 15
  consistency of, during labor, 62
  dilation of, during labor, 62
  dysplasia of, 197–202
  effacement of, during labor, 62
  nerve supply, 15
  position of, during labor, 62
  postpartum changes in, 88
  softening and cyanosis ("cervical ripening"), 35
Cesarean delivery, 80
  infection following, 134
Chadwick's sign, 20
Chancroid, 241
Chandelier sign, 236
Chlamydia, 238
Chlamydia trachomatis, 236, 238
Chloasma, 33
Cholelithiasis and cholecystitis, during pregnancy, 109
Cholestasis, during pregnancy, 29
Choriocarcinoma, 232–233
Chorionic villus sampling (CVS), 49

Circumvillate placenta, 130
Clinical clerkship exam, preparing for, 5–7
  practice exams, 6
  tips for answering questions, 6–7
Clitoris, 14
Coagulation, during pregnancy, 31
Colon cancer screening, 262
Colostrum, 20, 90
Colposcopy with cervical biopsy and endocervical curettage, 201
Colpotomy, 161
Complete abortion, 139, 141
Condom
  female, 154
  male, 154
Condyloma acuminata (genital warts), 240–241
Cone biopsy and LEEP, 201–202
Congenital adrenal hyperplasias, 177
Constipation, during pregnancy, 29, 53
Contraception, 154–158
  barrier methods, 154–155
    cervical cap, 154–155
    condom, female, 154
    condom, male, 154
  hormonal agents, 155–157
    implantable, 157
    injectable, 156–157
    oral contraceptives, 155–156
  intrauterine device, 157–158
  postcoital/emergency, 158
Contraction stress test, during labor, 74
Cordocentesis, 49,51
Cornu, 15
Corpus, of uterus, 15
Corpus luteum cyst, 193–194
Corticosteroids
  effects during pregnancy, 33
  use in preterm labor, 123
Corticotropin-releasing hormone (CRH), 40
Cortisol and other corticosteroids, during pregnancy, 26, 42
CRH. *See* Corticotropin-releasing hormone
Cryotherapy, for cervical dysplasia, 202
Cushing syndrome/disease, 176–177

CVS. *See* Chorionic villus sampling

Cyst of canal of Nuck, 247

Cystocele, 256, 257, 258
  surgical repair of, 258

D

Delivery, standard method of, 70–72
  dystocia, 72
  episiotomy, 71
  hemostasis, postdelivery, 72
  nuchal cord, checking for, 70
  placenta, delivery of, 72
  placental separation, 71
  postdelivery tasks, 71
  shoulders, delivery of, 70
  uterine exam, postdelivery, 71
  vaginal lacerations, 70–71

Delivery note, sample, 9

Diabetes mellitus, during pregnancy, 104–106

Diastolic murmurs, during pregnancy, 29

DIC. *See* Disseminated intravascular coagulation

Diet, during pregnancy, 51

Dilation of cervix, during labor, 62

Discharge orders post–cesarean section, sample, 10

Disseminated intravascular coagulation (DIC), 144–145

Domestic violence, 270–271
  assessment of, 270
  reaction to, 270–271
  recognition of occurrence of, 270

Down syndrome (trisomy 21), 47

Drug use in pregnancy, 98–99
  amphetamines, 99
  cocaine, 98–99
  hallucinogens, 99
  marijuana, 98
  opiates, 99

Dysgerminoma, 221

Dyspareunia, 189

E

Eclampsia, 117, 145

Ectocervix, 15

Ectopic pregnancy, 141–143

Edwards syndrome (trisomy 18), 47

Effacement of cervix, during labor, 62

Eisenmenger syndrome, 100, 108

Elective (induced) abortion, 141, 148

Embryology, 37–38

Employment, during pregnancy, 54

End-of-life decisions, 272

Endocervical canal, 15

Endocervical curettage, 181, 201

Endocrine system, during pregnancy, 32–33
  adrenal gland, 32
  disorders, 104
    diabetes mellitus, 104–106
  pancreas, 33
  parathyroid glands, 32
  pituitary gland, 32
  plasma proteins, 33
  thyroid gland, 32

Endodermal sinus tumor, 221

Endometrial biopsy, 165, 181

Endometrial cancer, 211–215
  clinical presentation, 212
  general facts, 212
  grading, 214
  hyperplasia, 213
  postmenopausal bleeding, differential diagnosis of, 212–213
  staging of, 214
  treatment of, 215
  uterine sarcoma, 215
  workup for, 213–214
    histologic subtypes, 214

Endometriosis, 164, 184, 187–190, 192
  adenomyosis vs., 190

Endometritis, 134

Endometrium, 16

Energy requirements, during pregnancy, 24, 25

Enterocele, 257, 258
  Moschovitz repair, 258

Enzyme-linked immunosorbent asay (ELISA), 240

Epidural analgesia, 85

Epilepsy, and pregnancy, 106–107

Episiotomy, infection following, 134

Erythroblastosis fetalis, 47

Erythrocyte sedimentation rate (ESR), during pregnancy, 26, 31

Estradiol, 42, 172

Estriol, 42, 47

Estrogen effects, during pregnancy, 33

Estrogen replacement therapy, 251, 252

Estrone, 42

Ethics, 272–274
  end-of-life decisions, 272
  informed consent, 273
  life-sustaining treatment, 272
  office health maintenance tests, 274
  patient confidentiality, 273–274
  reproductive issues, 273

Exercise, during pregnancy, 52

External os, 15

F

Fallopian cell carcinoma, 223–224

Fallopian (uterine) tubes, 17
  blood supply, 17
  nerve supply, 17
  parts, 17

False labor (Braxton Hicks contractions), 59

Fasting insulin levels, during pregnancy, 26

Female genitalia, external, 14

Fetal death, 144

Ferning test, 61

Fertilization, 36

Fetal heart rate
  beat-to-beat variability, 77–78
  monitoring, 73
  patterns during labor, 75–78
  tachycardia, 77

Fetal heart tones (FHTs), 22

Fetal imaging, 48–51
  amniocentesis, 49
  chorionic villus sampling (CVS), 49
  cordocentesis, 49, 51
  genetic testing, 51
  ultrasound, 48–49

Fetal lung maturity, assessing, 123

Fetal monitoring, continuous electronic, 73

Fetal skull, 61

Fetal vessel rupture, 129–30
  vasa previa, 129
  velamentous cord insertion, 129–130

Fetus, assessment of during labor, 63–68
  Leopold maneuvers, 63–65

Fetus, assessment of during labor
    (*continued*)
    fetal attitude and posture, 65
    fetal positions, 64
    lie, 63
    presentation/presenting part,
        63
    malpresentations, 65–68
        breech presentations, 66
        brow presentation, 66
        face presentation, 65
        shoulder dystocia, 66–68
        sinciput presentation, 66
    normal presentation (vertex), 65
Fitz-Hugh–Curtis syndrome, 238
Fluorescent *in situ* hybridization
    (FISH), 51
Follicle-stimulating hormone
    (FSH), 32
Fundal height, during pregnancy,
    20, 46
Fundus, 15

G

Gamete intrafallopian transfer
    (GIFT), 167
Gardnerella vaginalis, 236
Gastrointestinal system, during
    pregnancy, 29
    gallbladder, 29
    liver, 29
Genetic testing, 51
Genital herpes, 239–240
Genital warts (condyloma acumi-
    nata), 240–241
Genitourinary system, during preg-
    nancy, 29–30
    bladder, 30
    renal function, 30
    renal tubule changes, 30
    ureters, 30
Germinal epithelium, 17
Gestational age, assessment of,
    44–45
Gestational diabetes, 104–106
    effects of, 105
Gestational trophoblastic neopla-
    sia, 229–234
    choriocarcinoma, 232–233
    definition, 230
    hydatidiform mole, 230–232
        complete, 230
        invasive, 231–232
        partial, 230

placental site trophoblastic tu-
    mor (PSTT), 233–234
    treatment, 233, 234
    World Health Organization
        (WHO) prognostic scoring
        system, 233
Globulin, during pregnancy, 26
Glomerular filtration rate (GFR),
    during pregnancy, 25
Glucagon, during pregnancy, 26,
    33
Glucose tolerance test, 105
Gonadoblastomas, 178
Gonorrhea, 237
Granulosa–theca cell tumors, 178,
    223

H

Haemophilus ducreyi, 241
hCG. *See* Human chorionic go-
    nadotropin
Health maintenance and screening
    tools, 262–264
    bacteriuria testing/urinalysis, 264
    colon cancer screening, 262
    immunizations, 264
    laboratory testing, 262–263
        cholesterol, 262
        fasting glucose, 263
        lipids, 263
        thyroid-stimulating hormone
            (TSH), 262
    mammography, 262
    manual breast exams, 262
    Pap smear, 262
    sexually transmissible infection
        testing, 263
    tuberculosis (TB) skin testing,
        263
Heartburn (reflux esophagitis), dur-
    ing pregnancy, 29, 53
Heart rate, during pregnancy, 25
HELLP syndrome, during preg-
    nancy, 117
Hematologic changes during preg-
    nancy, 31
Hemoglobin concentration, during
    pregnancy, 31
Hemorrhoids, during pregnancy,
    29, 54
Hemosiderosis, 172
Hereditary nonpolyposis colon can-
    cer (HNPCC), 219

Herpes gestationis, 34
Hidradenomas, 247
High-density lipoprotein (HDL),
    during pregnancy, 27, 28
Hirsutism and virilism, 175–178
HIV. *See* Human immunodefi-
    ciency virus
Hormone replacement therapy,
    251–253
hPL. *See* Human placental lacto-
    gen
Human chorionic gonadotropin
    (hCG), 40, 47
Human immunodeficiency virus
    (HIV), 240
    and pregnancy, 107
    testing for, 263
Human papillomavirus (HPV),
    240–241
Human placental lactogen (hPL),
    40
Hydatidiform mole, 230–232
    complete, 230
    invasive, 231–232
    partial, 230
Hydrops tubae perfluens, 224
11β-Hydroxylase deficiency, 177
21-Hydroxylase deficiency, 177
Hyperemesis gravidarum, 20
Hyperprolactinemia, 173
Hypertensive diseases of preg-
    nancy, 116–119
    antihypertensive agents used,
        119
    chronic hypertension, 116
    eclampsia, 117
    HELLP syndrome, 117
    preeclampsia, 116–117
    transient hypertension, 116
Hyperthecosis, 177
Hypogastric artery, 15
Hypogastric plexus, 15
Hypoglycemic agents, use in preg-
    nancy, 103
Hypoxemia, 75
Hypoxia, 75
Hysterectomy, 161, 195, 205, 258
Hysterosalpingogram, 165

I

Immunizations, 264
    during pregnancy, 55
Impetigo herpetiformis, 34
Implantation, 36

In vitro fertilization (IVF) and embryo transfer, 166
Incomplete abortion, 138–139, 141
Induced abortion, 141, 147–149
  assessment of the patient, 148
  definition, 148
  methods of, 149
    less common, 149
  therapeutic, indications for, 148
  types of, 148
Inevitable abortion, 138, 141
Infections, perinatal 110
  bacterial, 112–113
  viral, 111–112
Infertility, 163–167
  assisted reproductive technologies, 166
    artificial insemination of donor sperm, 166
    definition, 166
    gamete intrafallopian transfer (GIFT), 167
    in vitro fertilization (IVF) and embryo transfer, 166
    intracytoplasmic sperm injection (ICSI), 166
    zygote intrafallopian transfer (ZIFT), 167
  definition, 164
  female factors affecting, 64
  internal architecture study, 165–166
    hysterosalpingogram, 165
    structural abnormalities, treatment for, 166
  laparoscopy, exploratory, 166
  ovulation, methods of assessing, 165
    possible causes and treatments of, 165
  workup for, 164–166
    abnormal sperm findings, treatment for, 165
    semen analysis, 164–165
Inflammatory bowel disease (IBD), 184
Informed consent, 273
Infundibulum, 17
Insulin sensitivity, during pregnancy, 24, 26, 33
Integumentary system/skin, during pregnancy, 33–34
  pruritic dermatologic disorders unique to pregnancy, 34

Internal os, 15
Intracytoplasmic sperm injection (ICSI), 166
Intramural part, of fallopian (uterine) tube, 17
Intrauterine device, 157–158
Isthmus, 17

J

Joint changes, during pregnancy, 24

K

Kallmann syndrome, 172
Karyotyping, 51
Kleihauer–Bettke test, 47, 125
Kleine regnung, 180

L

Labia majora, 14
Labor
  abnormalities of third stage of, 130–133
    abnormal placentation, 131–132
    macrosomia, 132–133
    postpartum hemorrhage, immediate, 130–131
    uterine inversion, 132
  amniotic fluid index during, 74–75
  arrest of, 72
  assessment of, 60–61
  biophysical profile, 74
  cardinal movements of, 68–69
    descent, 68
    engagement, 68
    expulsion, 69
    extension, 68–69
    external rotation (restitution), 69
    flexion, 68
    internal rotation, 68
  clinical signs of, 60
    bloody show, 60
    rupture of membranes (ROM), 60
  contraction stress test during, 74
  and delivery
    pain control during, 82–85
  fetal heart rate monitoring during, 73
  induction of, 79–80

  confirmation of term, 79
  contraindications, 79
  indications, 79
  induction methods, 80
  maternal vital signs during, 73
  nonstress test (NST) during, 74
  patterns, abnormal, 78, 79
  preterm, 119–123
  three stages of, 58–59
    first stage, 58–59
    second stage, 59
    third stage, 59
  true vs. false (Braxton Hicks contractions), 59
Laparoscopy, exploratory, 166
Laser therapy, for cervical dysplasia, 202
Leg cramps, during pregnancy, 54
Leiomyoma, 184, 194–195
Leopold maneuvers, 63–65
Leutinizing hormone (LH), 32
Lichen planus, 246
Lichen sclerosis, 246
Lichen simplex chronicus (LSC), 246
Life-sustaining treatment, 272
Ligaments, of the pelvic viscera, 16
Linea nigra, 33
Lipids, during pregnancy, 27–28
Lipoprotein (a), during pregnancy, 27
Low-density lipoprotein (LDL), during pregnancy, 27, 28, 42
Luteoma of pregnancy, 178
Lymphogranuloma venereum, 238
Lynch II syndrome, 219

M

Macrosomia, 132–133
Mammography, 262
Manual breast exams, 262
Mastitis, 134
McRoberts maneuver, 67
Mean corpuscular volume (MCV), during pregnancy, 26
Meconium, 61
Melanocyte-stimulating hormone, 33
Melasma, 33
Menometrorrhagia, 180
Menopause, 249–253
  definitions, 250

Menopause *(continued)*
  factors affecting age of onset, 250
  physiology during the menopausal period, 251, 252
  physiology during the perimenopausal period, 250–251
  and sexual response, 267
  treatment of adverse effect of, 251–253
    estrogen replacement therapy, 251, 252
    hormone replacement therapy, 251–253
Menorrhagia, 180, 212
Menstruation, 169–178
  amenorrhea, 172–173
  androgen excess, hirsutism, and virilization, 175–178
  development, 170
    puberty, 170
    precocious puberty, 170
  hyperprolactinemia, 173
  menstrual cycle, 170–172
    follicular phase, first part of, 170
    follicular (proliferative) phase, 171
    luteal phase, 172
    ovulation, 171–172
  premenstrual syndrome (PMS), 174–175
    premenstrual dysphoric disorder (PMDD), 175
  retrograde, 188
Mesometrium, 16
Metabolism, during pregnancy, 24, 28
Metrorrhagia, 180, 212
Mifepristone (RU 486), 272
Missed abortion, 139, 141
Mittelschmerz, 184
Mons pubis, 14
"Morning sickness," 53
Multiple gestation, 38, 47
Myomectomy, 195
Myometrium, 16

N

Naegele's rule, 45–46
Nausea, 20
  and vomiting, during pregnancy, 53

Neisseria gonorrhoeae, 236, 237
Neural tube defects (NTDs), 46
Neutrophils, during pregnancy, 26
Nitrazine test, 61
Nocturia, during pregnancy, 30
Nonstress test (NST), during labor, 74
Normal anatomy. *See* Anatomy, normal
Nutritional needs of the mother during pregnancy, 51–52
  diet, 51
  pica, 52
  vegetarians, 52
  vitamins, 51
  weight gain, 51

O

Obstetric admission history and physical, sample, 7–9
Obstetrics and gynecology, awards for, 275–279
Obstetrics and gynecology clerkship, how to succeed in, 1–10
  behavior on the wards, 2–4
  organize your learning, how to, 5
  prepare for the clinical clerkship exam, how to, 5–7
  sample delivery note, 9
  sample discharge orders post–cesarean section, 10
  sample obstetric admission history and physical, 7–9
  sample post–cesarean section note, 10
  sample post-NSVD discharge orders, 10
  sample postpartum note, 9
  terminology, 7
Oligohydramnios, 75
Oligomenorrhea, 172, 180
Oral contraceptives, 155–156
Orgasmic disorder, 268–269
Os, cervical, 15
Ovarian cancer, 217–224
  epidemiology, 218
  epithelial cell, 218
    CA-125, 218
    clinical presentation, typical, 218
    histologic subtypes, 218
    protective factors, 219
    risk factors, 218–219

fallopian cell carcinoma, 223–224
hereditary syndromes, 219
nonepithelial, 221
  histologic types, 221–223
staging of, 219, 220
treatment of, 20–221
  poor prognostic indicators, 221
  postoperative management, 220–221
workup, 219
  screening recommendations, 219
Ovarian cyst, 192
  functional, 193–194
    follicular, 193
    lutein, 193–194
  ruptured, 185
Ovarian failure, premature, 172
Ovarian germ cell tumors (GCTs), 221–223
Ovarian sex cord–stromal tumors, 223
Ovaries, 17
  blood supply, 17
  histology, 17
  nerve supply, 17
Ovulation, 36, 171–172
  and chronic pelvic pain, 184
  methods of assessing, 165
  possible causes and treatments of, 165
Oxytocin, 80

P

Pain control, during labor and delivery, 82–85
  analgesia and sedation, 83
  anesthesia, 83
    general, 83
    regional, 83–85
  lower genital tract innervation, 83
  nonpharmacological methods of, 83
Pap smear, 181, 198–200, 262
Papular dermatitis, 34
Paracervical block, 84
Parathyroid glands, 32
Patient confidentiality, 273–274
Pediculosis pubis (crabs), 241
Pelvic inflammatory disease (PID), 184, 236–237

Pelvic masses, 191–195
  diagnostic tests for causes of, 192
  differential diagnoses, 192
  leiomyomas (fibroids), 194–195
  ovarian cysts, functional, 193–194
    follicular, 193
    lutein, 193–194
Pelvic nerve, 15
Pelvic pain, 183–186
  acute, 185
  chronic, 184–185
Pelvic relaxation, 255–260
  anatomy of pelvic floor support, 256
  prolapse, 256–258
  urinary incontinence, 259–260
Pelvic types, 86
Pelvic viscera, ligaments of, 16–17
Perinatal infections, 110
  bacterial, 112–113
  viral, 111–112
Pfanensteil incision, 81
Pica, 52
Pituitary gland, 32
Pituitary stalk compression, 172
Placenta, 38
  circumvallate, 130
Placenta accreta, 131–132
Placenta increta, 131–132
Placenta percreta, 131–132
Placenta previa, 128–129
Placental abruption (abruptio placentae), 127–128, 145
Placental site trophoblastic tumor (PSTT), 233–234
  treatment, 233, 234
  World Health Organization (WHO) prognostic scoring system, 233
Placentation, 36, 38
  abnormal, 131–132
Plasma aldosterone, during pregnancy, 26
Plasma cholesterol, during pregnancy, 27
Plasma prolactin, during pregnancy, 26
Plasma proteins, 33
Plasma volume, during pregnancy, 26, 31
Platelet reactivity, during pregnancy, 31

Polycystic ovarian syndrome (PCOS), 172, 173, 177, 180, 212
Polyhydramnios, 75
Polymenorrhea, 180
Portio vaginalis, 15
Post–cesarean section note, sample, 10
Postcoital bleeding, 182
Post-NSVD discharge orders, sample, 10
Postimplantation, 38
Postmenopausal bleeding, 181–182
  differential diagnosis of, 212–213
Postpartum care, routine, 90–92
  first few days, 91–92
    abdominal wall relaxation, 92
    bowel function, 91
    diet, 92
    discomfort/pain management, 92
    immunizations, 92
  first several hours, 91
    bladder function, 91
    care of the vulva, 91
    early ambulation, 91
  immediately after labor, 90–91
  maternal follow-up care, 94–95
    breast-feeding, 94–95
  psychiatric disorders, 95–96
    maternity/postpartum blues, 95
    postpartum depression, 95
    postpartum psychosis, 96
Postpartum hemorrhage, immediate, 130–131
Postpartum infection, 133–134
  types of, 134
Postpartum note, sample, 9
Postpartum patient education, 92–93
  coitus, 93
  discharge, 93
  infant care, 93
  lactational amenorrhea method of contraception, 93
  oral contraceptives, 93
Precocious puberty, 170
Preeclampsia, 116–117, 145
Pregnancy
  antepartum, 43–56
    abdominal exam and fundal height, 46

    answers to commonly asked questions, 52–56
    emergency situations during, 56
    fetal imaging, 48–51
    gestational age, assessment of, 44–45
    nutritional needs of the mother during, 51–52
    prenatal care, 44
    Rh incompatibility and pregnancy, 47–48
    serum screening, maternal, 46–47
  complications of, 115–134
    abnormalities of third stage of labor, 130–133
    hypertensive diseases, 116–119
    postpartum infection, 133–134
    premature rupture of membranes, 123–125
    preterm labor, 119–123
    third-trimester bleeding, 125–130
  conception, 36–39
    developmental ages, 38
    fertilization, 36
    implantation, 36
    multiple gestation, 38
    ovulation, 36
    placenta, 38
    placentation, 36, 38
    postimplantation, 38
    preimplantation, 36
  contraindications to, 100
  diagnosis of, 19–22
    β-hCG, 21–22
    fetal heart tones (FHTs), 22
    history, 20
    signs, 20
    symptoms, 20
    ultrasonic scanning (US), 22
  ectopic, 141–143
  intrapartum, 57–86
    cardinal movements of labor, 68–69
    cervical exam during, 62
    cesarean delivery, 80
    clinical signs of labor, 60
    delivery, standard method of, 70–72

Pregnancy (*continued*)
  fetal heart rate patterns during, 75–78
  fetus, assessment of, 63–68
  high-risk patients, management of, 73–75
  induction of labor, 79–80
  labor, three stages of, 58–59
  laboring patient, assessment of, 60–61
  labor patterns, abnormal, 78, 79
  low-risk patients, management of, 72–73
  pain control during labor and delivery, 82–85
  true labor vs. false labor, 59
  uterus, blood facts about, 59
  vaginal birth after cesarean delivery (VBAC), 81–82
  luteoma of, 178
  medical conditions and infections in, 97–113
    acute abdomen, 109
    cardiovascular disease, 107–108
    endocrine disorders, 104–106
    epilepsy, 106–107
    HIV, 107
    perinatal infections, 110
    pulmonary disease, 108–109
    renal and urinary tract disorders, 109
    social risk factors, 98–100
  normal anatomical adaptations in, 35–36
    uterus, 35–36
    vagina, 35
  nutritional recommendations in, 100
  physical activity recommendations in, 100
  physiology of, 23–42
    cardiovascular system, 28–29
    central nervous system, 28
    changes in the body during pregnancy, 25–27
    endocrine system, 32–33
    gastrointestinal system, 29
    general effects on the mother, 24
    genitourinary system, 29–30
    hematologic, 31
    integumentary system/skin, 33–34

respiratory system, 28
postpartum, 87–96
  maternal follow-up care, 94–95
  patient education, 92–93
  psychiatric disorders, 95–96
  puerperium of normal labor and delivery, 88–90
proteins of, 39–40
steroids of, 39, 41, 42
teratology and drugs in, 100–104
Preimplantation, 36
Premature ovarian failure, 172
Premature rupture of membranes (PROM), 123–125
Premenopausal bleeding, abnormal, 180–181
  anovulatory, 180
  ovulatory, 180–181
Premenstrual syndrome (PMS), 174–175
  premenstrual dysphoric disorder (PMDD), 175
Prenatal care, 44
Preterm labor, 119–123
  risk, 120–122
Preventive health information, 264–265
Progesterone, 42, 172
Progestin challenge test, 172
Prolactin, 32, 40
PROM. *See* Premature rupture of membranes
Prostaglandins, 80
Proteins, during pregnancy, 26, 39–40
Prurigo gestationis, 34
Pruritic dermatologic disorders unique to pregnancy, 34
Pruritic urticarial papules and plaques of pregnancy (PUPPP), 34
Pruritus gravidarum, 34
Pseudomenopause, 190
Psoriasis, 246
Psychiatric disorders, postpartum, 95–96
  maternity/postpartum blues, 95
  postpartum depression, 95
  postpartum psychosis, 96
Psychotropics, 103
  antidepressants, 103
  tranquilizers, 103

Puberty, 170
  precocious, 170
  secondary sex characteristics, 170
  Tanner stages, 170
Pudendal arteries, 14
Pudendal block, 83–84
Puerperium of normal labor and delivery, 88–90
  blood, changes in, 90
  body weight, changes in, 90
  breast, changes in, 89
    colostrum, 90
    mature milk and lactation, 90
    milk, development of, 89
    milk-secreting machinery, development of, 89
  cervix and lower uterine segment, changes in, 88
  peritoneum and abdominal wall, 89
  placental site involution, 88
  urinary tract changes in, 89
  uterine changes, 88
    endometrial changes, 88
    involution of the uterine corpus, 88
  uterine vessels, changes in, 88
  vagina and vaginal outlet, changes in, 88
Pulmonary disease, and pregnancy, 108–109
  asthma, 108
  pulmonary embolism, 108–109
Pulmonary hypertension, 100, 108
Pyelonephritis, and pregnancy, 109

R

Rape, 271–272
Rape-related post-traumatic stress disorder (RR-PTSD), 271–272
Rectocele, 257, 258
Recurrent spontaneous abortion, 139, 141
Red blood cell (RBC) mass, during pregnancy, 26, 31
Reflux esophagitis (heartburn), during pregnancy, 29
Reiter syndrome, 238
Renal function, during pregnancy, 30

Renal plasma flow, during pregnancy, 26
Renal tubule changes, during pregnancy, 30
Reproductive history, terminology of, 44
Respiratory system, during pregnancy, 28
Rh incompatibility, and pregnancy, 47–48
    fetal danger due to, 48
    screening, 48
    sensitization, 47
    sensitized Rh-negative patient, management of, 48
    unsensitized Rh-negative patient, management of, 48
RhoGAM, 45, 48, 139
Round ligament, 17, 35
    pain, 54
RU 486 (mifepristone), 272
Rupture of membranes (ROM), 60

S

Safer sex practices, 266
Sample delivery note, 9
Sample discharge orders post–cesarean section, 10
Sample obstetric admission history and physical, 7–9
Sample post–cesarean section note, 10
Sample postpartum note, 9
Sample post-NSVD discharge orders, 10
Savage syndrome, 172
Schiller–Duval bodies, 221
Seat belt use, 265
Semen analysis, 164–165
    abnormal sperm findings, treatment for, 165
Septic abortion, 139–140
Sertoli–Leydig cell tumors, 178, 221, 223
Serum alkaline phosphatase, during pregnancy, 26
Serum screening, maternal, 46–47
    alpha-fetoprotein, maternal serum (MSAFP), 46–47
    estriol, 47
    human chorionic gonadotropin (hCG), 47

Sexual assault, 271–272
    rape-related post-traumatic stress disorder (RR-PTSD), 271–272
Sexual dysfunction, disorders of, 267–269
    orgasmic disorder, 268–269
    sexual arousal disorder, 268
    sexual desire disorders, 268
    sexual pain disorders, 269
Sexual relations, during pregnancy, 54
Sexual response and expression, female, 266–267
    adolescence, 266
    hormonal changes, 267
    menopause, 267
    menstrual cycle, 267
    postpartum, 267
    pregnancy, 267
    resolution, 266
    response cycle, 266
Sexually transmitted diseases, 235–241
    acquired immune deficiency syndrome (AIDS), 240
    chancroid, 241
    chlamydia, 238
    genital herpes, 239–240
    gonorrhea, 237
    human immunodeficiency virus (HIV), 240
    testing for, 263
    human papillomavirus (HPV), 240–241
    pediculosis pubis (crabs), 241
    pelvic inflammatory disease (PID), 236–237
    syphilis, 238–239
    testing for, 263
    toxic shock syndrome, 243
    vaginitis, 242–243
Sheehan syndrome, 172
Shoulder dystocia, 66–68
Skene's duct cyst, 247
Skin/integumentary system, during pregnancy, 33–34
    pruritic dermatologic disorders unique to pregnancy, 34
Spinal (subarachnoid) block, 84
Spontaneous abortion, 136–137
    chromosomal abnormalities and, 136

endocrine abnormalities and, 137
environmental factors and, 137
immunologic factors and, 137
infectious agents and, 136
uterine abnormalities and, 137
Squamocolumnar junction (SCJ), 198
Sterilization, 159–161
    colpotomy, 161
    hysterectomy, 161
    luteal phase pregnancy, 160
    tubal obstruction, 159–160
        complications of, 161
        hysteroscopic (essure), 159–160
        laparoscopic, 159
        reversibility of, 160
        salpingectomy, partial or total, 160
    vasectomy, 159
Steroids, of pregnancy, 39, 41, 42
Stress incontinence, during pregnancy, 30
Stroke volume, during pregnancy, 25
Substance abuse, 265
    alcohol, 265
    cigarettes, 265
Syncope, during pregnancy, 28
Syphilis, 238–239
Systemic vascular resistance, during pregnancy, 25
Systolic ejection murmurs, during pregnancy, 29

T

Tanner stages, 170
Teratogenic substances, common, 101–102
Teratology and drugs in pregnancy, 100–104
    analgesics, 103–104
    antiasthmatics, 104
    antibiotics and anti-infective agents, 104
    anticoagulants, 102
    cardiovascular drugs, 104
    common teratogenic substances, 101–102
    embryological age and teratogenic susceptibility, 100
    FDA pregnancy drug categories, 102, 103

Teratology and drugs in pregnancy (*continued*)
 hypoglycemic agents, 103
 psychotropics, 103
  antidepressants, 103
  tranquilizers, 103
Teratoma, of ovary, 222
Terminology, 7
Theca lutein cyst, 177, 194
Therapeutic (induced) abortion, 141, 148
 indications for, 148
Third-trimester bleeding, 125–130
 circumvillate placenta, 130
 extrusion of cervical mucus ("bloody show"), 130
 fetal vessel rupture, 129–30
  vasa previa, 129
  velamentous cord insertion, 129–130
 placenta previa, 128–129
 placental abruption (abruptio placentae), 127–128
 uterine rupture, 130
Threatened abortion, 138, 141
Thyroid gland, 32
Thyroid-stimulating hormone (TSH), 262
Thyroxine-binding globulin, during pregnancy, 27
Tidal volume, during pregnancy, 25, 28
Tobacco use in pregnancy, 98
Tocolytic therapy, 119, 122
Total body water, during pregnancy, 24, 25
Toxic shock syndrome, 243
Travel, during pregnancy, 55
Treponema pallidum, 238
Triglycerides, during pregnancy, 27, 28
Trisomy 18 (Edwards syndrome), 47
Trisomy 21 (Down syndrome), 47
Tubal obstruction, 159–160
 complications of, 161
 hysteroscopic (essure), 159–160
  Irving method, 160
  Kroener method, 160
  Madlener method, 160
  Parkland method, 160
  Pomeroy method, 160
  Uchida method, 160
 laparoscopic, 159

reversibility of, 160
salpingectomy, partial or total, 160
Tuberculosis (TB) skin testing, 263
Tubo-ovarian abscess, 192
Tunica albuginea, 17
Turner syndrome, 172

U

Ultrasonic scanning (US)
 for diagnosing pregnancy, 22
 fetal imaging, 48–49
 limitations, 22
Urinary frequency, during pregnancy, 30
Urinary incontinence, 259–260
 treatment of, 260
Urinary stasis, 29
Urinary tract infection, postpartum, 134
Uterine bleeding, abnormal, 179–182
 definitions, 180
 postmenopausal, 181–182
 premenopausal, abnormal, 180–181
  anovulatory, 180
  ovulatory, 180–181
Uterine contractions
 during labor, monitoring of, 72
 during pregnancy, 27
Uterine inversion, 132
Uterine sarcoma, 215
Uterine vessels, changes in during labor and delivery, 88
Uterosacral ligaments, 17
Uterus, 15–16
 blood facts about, 59
 blood supply, 16
 components, 15
 histology, 16
 monitoring activity of during labor, 72–73
 nerve supply, 16
 normal anatomical adaptations in pregnancy, 35–36
  cervix, 35
  isthmus, 36
  prolapse of, 258
  round ligament, 35
  vascular supply, 35
 placental site involution, 88
 postpartum changes in, 88
  endometrial changes, 88

involution of the uterine corpus, 88
rupture of, during pregnancy, 130

V

Vagina
 blood supply, 15
 clear cell adenocarcinoma of cervix and, 210
 nerve supply, 15
 postpartum changes in, 88
 vestibule of, 14
Vaginal birth after cesarean delivery (VBAC), 81–82
 candidates for, 81
 contraindications to, 81
 forceps delivery, 81
 vacuum delivery, 82
Vaginal cancer, 227–228
 diagnosis, 228
 signs and symptoms, 228
 staging of, 228
 treatment of, 228
Vaginal exam, during labor, 60–61, 73
Vaginitis, 242–243
Varicosities, during pregnancy, 53
Vasa previa, 129
Vasectomy, 159
Vegetarians, and pregnancy, 52
Velamentous cord insertion, 129–130
Venous dilation, during pregnancy, 29
Vernix, 61
Vertex (occipital) presentation, of fetus, 65
Very low-density lipoprotein (VLDL), during pregnancy, 27, 28
Vestibular bulb, 14
Vestibulitis, 246–247
Violence, exposure to during pregnancy, 99–100
Virilism, 175–178
Vital capacity, during pregnancy, 25, 28
Vitamins, during pregnancy, 51
Vulva, 14
 blood supply, 14
 lymph, 14
 nerve supply, 14

Vulvar disorders, 245–247
  cysts, 247
    of canal of Nuck, 247
    Bartholin's abscess, 247
    hidradenomas, 247
    sebaceous, 247
    Skene's duct, 247
  dystrophies, 246
    lichen planus, 246
    lichen sclerosis, 246
    lichen simplex chronicus
      (LSC), 246
  psoriasis, 246
  vestibulitis, 246–247
Vulvar dysplasia and cancer,
  225–228
  staging of, 227
  vaginal cancer, 227–228
  vulvar intraepithelial neoplasia
    (VIN), 226

W

Weight gain, during pregnancy, 24,
  25, 51

Western blot, 240
"Whiff" test, 243
White blood cell count, during
  pregnancy, 31
Woods corkscrew maneuver, 68
Wright's stain, 125

Z

Zavanelli maneuver, 68
Zygote intrafallopian transfer
  (ZIFT), 167